Glioblastoma
A guide for patients and loved ones

Your guide to glioblastoma and
anaplastic astrocytoma brain tumours

GIDEON BURROWS

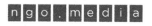

For Marie Hunter

Gideon Burrows was diagnosed with an incurable glioma brain tumour aged 35. He is a writer, bicycle mechanic, and lives close to the sea near Belfast, UK.

Also by the author

Living Low Grade: A patient guide to living with a slow growing brain tumour

This Book Will Not Cure Your Cancer

Chilli Britain: A Hot and Fruity Adventure

Men Can Do It: Why Dads Don't Do Childcare

The No-Nonsense Guide to the Arms Trade

Write for Charity

The Ethical Careers Guide

Martin and Me

Leo

Contents

Introduction

I WAS BROUGHT up on the outskirts of the Black
Country in England, so called because at one time it
was the industrial heart of the country and everything
was frequently covered in soot. By the time I was born
in 1977, the soot had gone. The factories and coal
mines across the broad industrial expanse of my home
town of Wolverhampton had long come to a halt.
Little had been left for the people once employed in
those industries.

I went to secondary school in a large village called
Wombourne, a well-to-do suburb where industrial
Wolverhampton gave way to the greenbelt. A few miles
further and the wonderful open valleys of Shropshire
and the hilly winding stretches of the Welsh
countryside take over.

It was at school, and later at sixth form college,
that I studied alongside Duncan Weaver. I do not
remember him well, though our families and those of
our friends must have moved in the same social circles.
After school our lives went in radically different

directions. Duncan eventually moved to the Netherlands, while I went from Wolverhampton to London. Eventually I crossed the sea too, but in another direction, to Ireland.

Our paths were not to cross again until 2013 when I began to write my first brain tumour book, *Brain Tumours: Living Low Grade*. Like me, Duncan had been diagnosed with a low grade brain tumour. He'd heard about my project from The Brain Tumour Charity, a UK organisation, and was a reader of my blog. He really wanted to contribute.

His story was so familiar to mine that it became a key part of the book. He had lots to share about his initial diagnosis of a low grade astrocytoma, his fears for the future, but mainly about the difficulties of dealing with the daily symptoms of a chronic disease. Both of us had learned to live low grade. We kept in touch frequently, and continued to check in when times got tough, comparing our experiences by email.

In November 2014, a year after we'd been reunited by our brain tumours, Duncan emailed me with the news. His tumour had taken a turn for the worse. It was no longer low grade; he had an anaplastic astrocytoma. A high grade tumour. The tumour had become malignant.

In 2012, the year London hosted the Olympic Games just down the road from my old home, I was diagnosed with a brain tumour. One that is inoperable, and will eventually end my life.

I am a writer. For all of my working life, I've been helping charities and good causes to get their message across more effectively through the written word. My natural response, even in the very earliest days of my diagnosis, was to get it down on paper. I started by making little notes, but that soon turned into a regular blog that charted my emotional and physical journey.

Some brain tumour patients want to know nothing of their diagnosis: not the type, not the nature of their illness, nor their predicted treatment, nor survival rates. I was exactly the opposite. I wanted to know everything.

What I discovered from researching my particular type of brain tumour – then a low grade oligodendroglioma – was that there was actually very little patient friendly information available about brain tumours. Information from hospitals and doctors tended to be technical and over medicalised. Information from charities was too general for my palate, and often over washed with emotive language which may be good for fundraising but can sometimes get in the way of understanding.

As I got to know the 'brain tumour community' it became clear there were many of us living low grade who similarly felt that the information we craved just didn't exist. We weren't hearing the stories of others like us. We weren't getting the medical information we needed about our situation.

By the time I had a biopsy in May 2013, I had decided to write a book about my type of brain tumour. I appealed for stories from other low grade brain tumour patients, and was overwhelmed by the response. People wanted to tell their own stories. I was merely the scribe, sewing together the stories of more than 20 patients and their families, recounting how their tumours had affected their lives, and providing medical and health information where it was relevant.

Brain Tumours: Living Low Grade became probably

one of the most used resources for low grade brain tumour patients in the UK, and it has sold across the world. It clearly met its intended aim: to fill an information gap, to support those desperate for answers to their questions: What? Why? What next? Patients and their families welcomed the straight talking, layperson's approach: I received so many emails from readers who said things like 'that's exactly how it was for me', 'you're so right', 'I have the same seizures', 'I have the same feelings of guilt/fear/joy/sadness'.

But there was another type of response that I received from many dozens of correspondents. These were people who hadn't had experience of a low grade glioma brain tumour. Theirs was a high grade brain tumour. One that was more immediately life threatening; one that demanded more urgent action than low grade brain tumours typically do. They were crying out for a book that they could use to inform themselves, and to help their families understand. They wanted the hard information and useful stories that *Brain Tumours: Living Low Grade* had provided for low grade patients.

Despite high grade brain tumours like glioblastomas and anaplastic astrocytomas being far more common in adults than low grade gliomas, no overarching information source was doing the job. Something was wanted and needed to put adult patients in the know, and in charge of their own brain tumour journey. Something was needed to help recently bereaved families to understand and come to terms with what had just happened.

For a long time, I believed the author of that book could not be me. I do not have a glioblastoma brain tumour. I do not have an astrocytoma brain tumour. Mine is a close cousin of the astrocytoma. It is life threatening and will most likely end my life, but it does not have the same profile or outlook as the previous two. As I write, my tumour is considered a high grade brain tumour, but my survival outlook is still measured in many many years, not months. Without specific experience of glioblastoma or anaplastic astrocytoma, I didn't feel close enough to these brain tumours to be able to step up to the plate.

And then something awful began to happen. Low grade astrocytoma patients who had featured in *Living Low Grade* as 'getting on with their life', resolutely dealing with the poor luck life had dealt them, began to transform into high grade patients. Friends and contributors who had 'astrocytoma Grade II' written next to their names in the book began to tell me their tumour had progressed to Grade III or IV. They wanted to tell me the new chapters of their stories. To the breaking of my heart, some of them began to die.

My story of low grade patients struggling to live with their brain tumours began to feel unfinished. My commitment to my original contributors was not yet over. The need to assist and support brain tumour patients with glioblastomas and high grade astrocytomas, and their families, remained. I had the capacity, the contacts, the ability and the knowledge to tell that story.

What does this book aim to do?

This book is a guide to adult glioblastoma and anaplastic astrocytoma for patients and their loved ones. The two brain tumours that are considered to have short life expectancies, and life changing effects before, during and after any treatment. Through offering basic medical information about brain cancer, as well as information about treatment options, prognosis and impact, I hope to help those affected to understand these brain tumours as best they can.

I hope to arm you with information that will form the basis for further research, for questions to oncologists, surgeons, doctors and support organisations. And I hope to illustrate, as best I can, what life and perhaps death can be like with these brain tumours.

Some of what I have to share, and the very real and generously shared stories of others who have been affected, you will find helpful. Some you won't. Some information you may know, much you will not. There are parts that some of you may not wish to know or face, while others will crave every word on every page. Whatever you take away from this book, I hope to provide you with some support, knowledge and empowerment.

You will hear it a hundred times: No two patients are the same. No two brain tumours are the same – not the same size, nor in the same place, nor will they cause the same symptoms, or respond to treatment in the same way. With that proviso in mind, I hope this book gives patients and their families some structure to the unimaginable and the unknown. Striking the balance giving readers enough information without overloading them, while trying neither to be too general nor too specific, is one of the key challenges I've faced.

Like *Brain Tumours: Living Low Grade* this book is most of all a collection of stories. It does not aim to, nor should it be taken as, a replacement for sound medical advice from your doctors, oncologists and other experts. Brain tumour research moves quickly, and just as two brain tumours are not the same, nor are two doctors, nor their opinions on your particular brain tumour. Everything you read here should be with that in mind: there are very few certainties in brain tumours, I am just attempting to paint a helpful picture.

Nor is this a cancer memoir, though it certainly contains a lot of memories. It is not a guide book, though some may find it helpful to find their way. It is an attempt to gather together wisdom and experience, with relevant medical information.

I hope that in experience, knowledge and understanding will rest some comfort and some ability to comprehend, and where relevant make choices. I hope the book will give you the chance to cry, to laugh, to hope and to prepare for the worst. In my experience, all are natural. All are healthy.

I cannot pretend that glioblastoma and anaplastic astrocytomas are not serious brain tumours. They are very serious. But as you come to properly understand them, you should beware of sensational headlines beloved of tabloid newspapers, particularly when a celebrity is involved, about 'deadly brain tumours', 'killer brain cancer' and 'brains riddled with cancer'.

The reality is far more subtle, far more nuanced and most often less brutal that such articles imply. Glioblastoma and anaplastic astrocytoma are not currently curable. That is a sad fact. But they are treatable. Let us try to start from there.

About these brain tumours

BY AGE 28, James Campling had found his perfect job. He was passionate about travelling. And the more adventurous the better. Becoming a nurse in the Royal Air Force meant he could travel all over the world. During his holidays, he would take further adventures, sometimes alone, sometimes with friends.

At the beginning of 2016, James spent Christmas in Mexico and Valentine's day hiking in Sudan. By May he was in India, visiting the tourist sights like the Taj Mahal and Delhi, but also going off the beaten track. Within 10 minutes of arriving at an Indian nature reserve, he found himself metres away from a wild tiger. Later that spring, he headed to Scandinavia, camping alone in the Finnish wilderness, following up with a trip to the Balkans.

Mobile phone signals never were very good on trains. Even less so in the extremely remote and desolate west of Finland. It was 15 June when the train James was travelling on went through a good signal spot. James' phone picked up a few missed calls from the same number. A number from his home dialling code, back in England.

It was his local doctor and James' stomach lurched as the railway tracks pitched the carriage from side to side. When he was able to connect, his doctor spoke quickly, precisely. She told him he had a brain tumour. James Campling's world, a world which had been full of endless possibilities, fell apart.

The next few pages may be a little complex, perhaps over technical. But they are necessary and I wanted to get them over with because they put the whole of the rest of what you will read in this book into context. It'll help you understand what, in the pages that follow, relates to the particular type of tumour you or a loved one has. And what does not.

Don't worry if some of the pages coming up seem a little opaque, as you go through the book as a whole you'll see some recurring patterns that will also chime with your own diagnosis. Forgive the necessary information dump I offer here, but I hope you'll understand. Take a deep breath, and off we go.

Astrocytoma and glioblastoma are from a group of brain tumours called gliomas, known because they grow from the glial cells in the brain. Glial cells are structural bits of the brain, a kind of glue or scaffold that surrounds and protects the nerve cells in the brain and spinal cord. They may also pass messages between nerve cells.

These brain tumours grow from a type of glial cell called astrocytes, the most frequently occurring cell in the brain. When the DNA in these astrocytes doesn't function correctly, the number of astrocytes growing – and others failing to die a natural cell death – gets out of control.

If these corrupted astrocytes grow very slowly, they are usually known as Grade I, called pilocytic astrocytoma, and are considered treatable and effectively curable, though they can create long term, life changing disability. These rarely occur in adults. In children, astrocytoma tumours are usually pilocytic astrocytoma.

If they grow slightly faster, and appear more abnormal under the microscope, they are considered Grade II astrocytomas. These tumours tend to be diffuse, meaning they infiltrate the brain as if they have tendrils weaving in and out of gaps between parts of the tissues. Someone shared with me the analogy of spilled ink infiltrating a sponge. For that reason, they can also referred to as 'diffuse astrocytoma'.

Low grade astrocytomas are usually treatable with surgery, radiotherapy and chemotherapy. But they almost always return. If they do return, they often come back as higher grade tumours. However, a patient can live for many years with an astrocytoma that is doing very little.

Grade II tumours are not really considered an emergency (unless they are causing some serious brain malfunction), though neither are they 'benign'. The term 'benign', once used frequently for these types of brain tumours, is now falling out of use. That's because the complications even the most inert brain tumour can cause in the brain cannot be said to be harmless, mainly because of the pressure they can put on the tissue surrounding them, and because they can cause a build up of brain fluid that causes harm.

When a corrupted astrocyte cell is very abnormal, growing quite rapidly and injuring healthy brain cells, the tumour is considered a Grade III or IV tumour. If Grade III it is known as an 'anaplastic astrocytoma'. If Grade IV it might be identified as a 'secondary glioblastoma'.

Glioblastomas can also appear *de novo*, meaning they are not understood to have ever been an astrocytoma previously. They're mostly made up of various different types of abnormal brain cells, with various genetic abnormalities, something which makes them harder to treat. This variety is called 'heterogeneity'. This type of tumour is known as 'primary glioblastoma'. They are considered the most malignant of brain tumours, and have the poorest prognosis. Unfortunately, they are also the most frequently occurring brain tumour in adults.

Only astrocytoma brain tumours can *become* glioblastomas, though other brain tumours can become Grade IV. (This book does not deal with them).

The difference between these different forms of astrocytoma and glioblastoma can be confusing, but their difference is relevant and important for reasons that become clear when we consider genetics and prognosis. The subtle difference between all of these tumours are explained in the table below.

General name	Description
Primary glioblastoma *de novo* (Grade IV)	A tumour which occurs with no apparent precursor tumour, made up of various cell types with various genetic mutations

Secondary glioblastoma (Grade IV)	A glioblastoma tumour that has emerged from/ still is an anaplastic astrocytoma
Anaplastic astrocytoma *de novo* (Grade III)	A high grade astrocytoma that does not appear to have been a lower grade astrocytoma
Anaplastic astrocytoma. (Grade III)	A high grade astrocytoma that is known to have transformed from a low grade astrocytoma
Astrocytoma, or diffuse astrocytoma (Grade II)	A lower grade brain tumour that may transform at some point into an anaplastic astrocytoma

The words 'primary' and 'secondary' here should not be confused with talk of primary and secondary tumours in cancer more generally. Outside of the specifics of the above, a *primary* brain tumour is one that has grown in the brain, with its origins as a brain cell.

A *secondary* brain tumour is one that has grown from cancerous cells that have migrated (metastasised) from elsewhere in the body, such as from breast, testicle or lung cells. Metastasised cancer cells remain abnormal versions of their original cell, so cannot become astrocytoma or glioblastoma tumours.

World Health Organization classification

In fact, it is easy to get confused about brain tumours and their grades in general. There are over 130 types of brain tumour, and various grades of each. This is one of the reasons why the World Health Organization (WHO) has moved away from a simple grading system to a far more comprehensive system of naming and recording brain tumours, based on their cell structure, activity, malignancy and genetic makeup. For many years to come, however, it is likely that the brain tumour community, including medics, will talk about brain tumours Grades I, II, III and IV.

For clarity in this book, you will find that I occasionally refer to a low or high grade, or Grade III and IV astroycytoma. But mostly I will talk about anaplastic astrocytomas and glioblastomas as that is the general direction of travel for naming and classification. You may have heard, or been diagnosed with, an oligoastrocytoma brain tumour. This is a tumour that has grown from a mix of oligodendrocytes and astrocytes. After many years of debate, WHO is currently classifying these tumours as one of the two, depending on the majority type of cell. Like astrocytomas, they too tend to be diffuse and come in both Grade II and Grade III forms. They are life threatening but are not often considered to be as malignant as astrocytomas.

WHO has identified that primary glioblastomas are made up of various types of brain cells with various genetic mutations, explaining further why identifying the exact genetic makeup of brain tumours is becoming more and more important in identifying the best treatment and prognosis.

Like our education, mine and Duncan Weaver's brain tumour journeys began in a very similar way. Mine had been in 2012 after a morning of pushing it hard on the bike while training with my cycling club. His had been during a vigorous game of five-a-side football among friends.

Both of us had what we could only describe as a 'funny turn'. Duncan had experienced dizziness on the football field, his limbs felt weird and his face felt numb. That was in November 2010. We both went to our GPs who referred us to a stroke clinic. They in turn referred us for a barrage of tests: blood flow, an ECG on our heart beats, blood tests, and an MRI.

It was possible, Duncan's doctor had said, he had a small hole in the heart. That could be fixed with a simple operation. Otherwise, it might be epilepsy. That would be controlled with medication. All in all, it was not too much to worry about. Duncan and Loes, his wife of just three months, pushed on with a long planned move: from the UK to the Netherlands. They celebrated New Year in their new home.

Three days later, Duncan flew back to the UK to see his stroke consultant again, taking his parents with him. Duncan had to tell his new wife by phone: *I have a brain tumour.*

The consultant asked Duncan to stay at the hospital for a few days, while they ran some more tests and his wife flew in to be with him. There were no other tumours in his body, so doctors confirmed they suspected Duncan had a low grade brain tumour. One that might be fatal one day, but for the time being was growing slowly, if at all. He was prescribed Epilim (sodium valproate), a long established anti-seizure drug.

He was told he shouldn't drive and was sent on his way. His treatment – the standard for low grade brain tumours at the time – would be to watch and wait.

The doctors were satisfied, but Duncan and Loes were not. They felt cheated that, after all the tests, the hospital stay and the diagnosis, the supposed solution was to do nothing. But after much research, they decided to put their faith in the hands of the specialists. For Duncan, he would have to get used to doing nothing. Nothing but watch and wait for the slow growing lump in his head to show its hand.

Occurrence

Anaplastic astrocytomas and glioblastomas are the fastest growing and most common form of brain tumour. Data about the occurrence of brain tumours worldwide are actually very hard to come by, and more specific data about very specific brain tumour types even harder. However, the following does give us at least an impression.

First, brain tumours as a whole, including anaplastic astrocytomas and glioblastomas, but also with other malignant brain tumours:

An estimated 24,790 new cases of primary malignant brain tumours were expected to be diagnosed in the US in 2016, according to the American Brain Tumor Association (ABTA).[1] There were around 11,000 new cases of brain or other central nervous system (CNS) tumours in the UK in 2014 according to Cancer Research UK – that's 30 cases diagnosed every day.[2]

Secondly, more specific to the brain tumours we are talking about, and according to the World Health

Organization (WHO):[3]

Glioblastoma is the most frequently occurring brain tumour. Around 45-50% of all primary malignant brain tumours are glioblastomas. Around nine out of ten of all glioblastomas are likely to be *primary glioblastomas*. Most of them will be in older people, and predominate in patients over 55 years old.

Around one in ten of all glioblastomas are likely to be *secondary glioblastoma/anaplastic astrocytoma*. These are more often found in younger patients.

Yet, with around just three to four of all kinds of glioblastoma tumours diagnosed per 100,000 people, across the Americas and Europe (men slightly more often than women), it is still considered a very rare form of cancer. Compare, for example, the 124.9 per 100,000 of women per year in the United States who will get breast cancer.[4] In eastern Asia brain cancer is even more rare, though those figures may be because of low reporting or recording rates.

Okay, that's the end of the major information dump. Let's see what all this really means.

What does malignant mean in brain tumours?

This was certainly one of the biggest questions I had when I was first diagnosed with a brain tumour. It wasn't clear whether the damage done by brain tumours was simply because they grew – and therefore put pressure on other parts of the brain in the confined space of the skull – or whether there was something else going on.

Primary glioblastomas usually grow rapidly. There can be less than three months between no obvious brain abnormality and a fully developed tumour.

Normally, brain cells multiply and then die off in a continuous cycle of renewal. But in brain tumours, those cells don't 'switch off' when old or damaged. They continue to live, as well as multiply into similarly abnormal cells, creating a tumour.

It is clear that pressure build up because of lack of space is a key reason why brain tumours of all kinds and grades are very dangerous. Cancer cells in the brain multiply quicker than normal cells. This 'squeezing' can cause normal brain cells to malfunction or stop functioning altogether, or cut off blood supply. They can also cause blockages in the usual pathways of fluid in the brain. The build up of pockets of cerebral fluid can cause this same kind of pressure. It's why surgery is often vital for removing as much tumour as possible to free up some space, and to drain off any build up of fluid.

But when a tumour becomes malignant there's more to it than that. Anaplastic astrocytoma and glioblastoma are malignant tumours. Not only do they grow rapidly, but their cells invade healthy brain tissue and destroy the cells there. Cancerous cells create their own blood vessels, further fuelling their own multiplication.

Since the brain, consciously and unconsciously, controls all of the body's functions, disrupted brain workings can affect our bodies, our mental capacity, and even the functions we take for granted such as breathing and heartbeat. The larger the tumour, and the more infused it is into healthy brain tissue, the likelier it is to have an impact. Eventually, a malfunctioning brain cannot keep the body or the mind alive.

Together, those behaviours classify malignant

tumours as brain cancer. In the UK, we don't tend to use that term. In the United States and elsewhere, the term 'brain cancer' is more readily used instead of, or as well as, brain tumour.

Astrocytoma and glioblastoma can cause cell death (necrosis) among the cells surrounding the tumours. The centres of these brain tumours often have large clumps of dead cells, space or fluid rather than healthy brain cells. Since these tumours tend to appear not as single lumps, like a lime or kiwi, but are instead diffuse, it is not difficult to understand how their growth and attack on healthy brain cells around them can be very rapid and complex.

The spaces that grow where brain cells have been killed off by brain cancer can also become a problem, as they can fill with water or brain fluid, crowding the skull and causing pressure pain and functionality problems. Doctors often have to drain this fluid, to reduce pressure in the brain.

Why are glioblastomas so hardy?

Glioblastomas are aggressive tumours and often appear resistant to treatment. Scientists are trying to find out why this is.

One theory is that glioblastomas are made up of lots of different types of cells, with various genetic abnormalities, called heterogeneity. One or even two forms of treatment just cannot successfully attack all these types of cells and stop them from multiplying. Therefore the tumour is extremely resistant.

Some researchers believe glioblastomas have their own stem cells, a type of cell which can turn into any other kind of cell that is needed. So even a brain tumour that once appeared to have been killed off can return, rejuvenated from the stem cells the tumour contains. Both theories, or the two combined, are convincing explanations of why a glioblastoma will continue to grow despite repeated surgery, radiotherapy and chemotherapy. Much recent research is concentrating on these areas to attempt to create new treatments that are more effective.

What causes brain tumours?

First things first. Your brain tumour is not your fault. Indeed, even if there was a lifestyle factor associated with brain tumours, it still would not be your fault. But there is no lifestyle factor. Or any other cause for brain tumours. There is nothing you could have done, or not done, or done differently, to prevent an anaplastic astrocytoma or glioblastoma from growing in your brain.

Many years of research has failed to clearly identify any cause of glioblastoma tumours. Not mobile phones. Not overhead power lines. Not TV signals. Not diet. Not obesity. Not even smoking.

People can get brain tumours at any age, with any lifestyle, from any race or ethnicity, of any gender and background. Naturally, the older the patient becomes the more likely they are to develop a brain tumour *in their lifetime*. That's simply because there are more years in their lives in which the chance of DNA mutation causing a brain tumour exists. The same applies to most cancers.

There is some evidence that there is an increased risk of brain tumours in adults who have had other types of cancers, but further research is needed to confirm this. Whether this is due to the cancer or treatment for that earlier cancer has not been established. It is clear that not having treatment for an early cancer is far more dangerous than the minute chance of developing some kind of brain tumour later on. This same rule applies to those who receive radiation for their brain tumour: There is a small chance it could cause a brain tumour in the distant future, but the benefit of treatment now far outweighs that chance.

A very small number of brain tumours are known to be related to hereditary conditions. While glioblastoma and astrocytoma are likely to be related to genetic malfunction, their malfunctioning genes are not regarded as inherited.

It is known that DNA disruption and mutation causes these brain tumours to develop. The latest research indicates some 26 genetic errors may be required to create a brain tumour. Research is gradually discovering which genes are involved.

In 70 to 80 percent of glioblastomas, according to The Brain Tumour Charity in the UK, the tumour is characterised by the loss of chromosome 10 and the genes it carries.[5] Broken down further, several genes appear to be involved in the initial development of glioblastomas. These include the checkpoint genes 'TP53', 'PTEN', 'NF1' and 'p16-INK4A', and growth stimulator genes 'EGFR' and 'PDGFRA'.

Don't worry, these codes mean nothing to me either. The point is that scientists are discovering that chromosomes and genes, our DNA, are intimately involved in causing brain tumours. But this doesn't explain *why* we get brain tumours. That's because it is far from known what causes the disruptions in these chromosomes and genes. Explaining tumour formation in terms of DNA is to tell only a tiny bit of the story, and brings us only a little closer to the answer to the question: *why do I have a brain tumour?*

As the ABTA concludes, 'Scientists are conducting environmental, occupational, familial and genetic research to identify common links among patients. Despite a great deal of research on environmental hazards, no direct causes have been found.'[6]

The sad truth is – as science currently understands it – most brain tumours just happen. They are the worst of luck. Unfortunately, scammers and misinformed do-gooders may try to tell you that diet, power lines or some other bogeyman is the cause of brain tumours, and that they have either the ultimate protection or cure. You should treat such claims with extreme caution.

Detecting brain tumours

LIAN DAVIS'S MUM, Gillian Handley, wasn't a moaner. In fact, she was the opposite: she was the one who would always listen to everyone else's problems. Gillian had had a difficult split with her husband, so Lian felt like her mum already knew about hurt. So she always wanted to ease it in other people. She wanted to take care and look after everybody.

She had been a foster parent. Helped women escaping domestic violence. She'd gone hungry to feed her children. She was generous with her time, her door was always open. What little she had she shared. She had a wicked sense of humour, often a little naughty. With her practical jokes, she'd often act like a teenager, not someone in her late 50s.

So when Gillian started complaining about headaches, it puzzled Lian. She was used to her mum just getting on with things, rarely complaining about anything. Her mum went to the doctors of course – dozens of times over two years – but she only ever came away with instructions to lose weight, or take another painkiller.

But the painkillers had long since stopped working. Lian's mum described the headaches not only as painful, but like her head had become super sensitive. When Lian brushed Gillian's hair, she'd complain her daughter was pulling too hard. Sometimes brushing her hair hurt her mum so much, she would get nauseous. Something wasn't right, but no-one suspected what was really happening. Why would they?

Signs and symptoms

There do not seem to be any statistics, or even estimates, about the signs or symptoms that lead doctors to first suspect their patients have a brain tumour. However, it is known that well over half in the UK are diagnosed after an emergency visit to hospital, for example after suffering some kind of seizure.[7]

In fact, brain tumours are really quite rare so it's very likely your doctor will have suspected something quite different before beginning to come around to the idea there might be a lump in your brain.

> "Ironically I was working both in medical screening and as a remedial personal trainer when I started experiencing nocturnal tonic clonic seizures and extended bouts of disorientation. A run of misdiagnosis followed whilst I slowly tore my muscles to pieces. Those eventually became waking seizures, and an MRI was finally brought to the table. I received an initial Grade II astrocytoma guestimate prior to surgery, which while successful in itself has since given way to an

anaplastic astrocytoma diagnosis."
Jack Webb

In my case, my doctor referred me to a stroke specialist, who tested my physical reactions, and to a sonographer, who measured the blood flow into my brain. Both were normal and it was only then I was referred on for imaging of the inside of my brain.

"My twin sister Sue Rossides' husband died in January 2016. She'd nursed him at the home the three of us shared in Greece. It was traumatic for her because they'd only been married 15 months. The night before his funeral she fell ill and I called our doctor. Her blood pressure was soaring, and we put it down to grief and stress. But she continued to feel unwell, and after blood tests was put on medication for an underactive thyroid. She kept describing her dizziness as different to normal, 'as if the floor is breaking up beneath my feet'. The sensation got worse and worse, until she couldn't walk around without holding onto the furniture. Then, one April morning, she called me from upstairs. I found her slumped across her desk, saying she'd got flashing lights in front of her eyes. The doctor came, and while he was there she had a massive seizure right in front of our eyes.

"An ambulance took her to hospital, and the doctors there told us she was in a critical condition. They were transferring her to another hospital in Greece for scans and further tests. By the time I was allowed to see her, she was awake and feeling strange, but with no memory of what had just happened. The doctors there diagnosed epilepsy, but transferred her again to the University Hospital two hours away. They did an MRI and told me that she had what looked like a massive infection in her brain.

"The next day the consultant called me into a private office whether they broke the news that they had 'found something'."
Joanna Waters, sister of Sue Rossides

Some brain tumour patients don't seem to have any symptoms at all, before suffering some total collapse from which they never recover. Others have very slowly growing symptoms, that almost imperceptibly get worse over time. Especially in older people, they can be mistaken for just 'getting old', being grumpy or perhaps the onset of dementia.

There are some key symptoms of brain tumours that do show themselves more clearly. By themselves, they may not have been thought relevant to brain tumours. But a few or more of them together really ought to be taken more seriously.

In each case, symptoms might last anything from 10 or 20 seconds, to many hours.

Seizures

A number of different occurrences may be called seizures. At one extreme are what most would call a full *grand mal* epileptic fit where the person has collapsed, is convulsing, perhaps biting their tongue and is unconscious. But there are also much milder physical seizures where the person is fully conscious, which may include involuntary movement, jerking, ticking, the rising of an arm or shoulder, a downturning of the mouth, or just a general feeling of being a bit absent.

> "The first thing I knew was waking up in a hospital bed in 1998. Completely out of the blue I had a couple of *grand mal* fits. Luckily I was teaching a couple of nurses at the time, so at least I was in a good place to have them. By the time I woke up I had had a CT scan that showed the tumour. We did not know any detail about it."
> Richard Stevens

> "I had a seizure on the plane I was working on as a flight attendant. It came totally out of the blue. One moment, I was setting up the galley and the next I had lost control of my eyes and blacked out when I hit the floor. Flight attendants go through training for this very situation, so I had three colleagues who knew exactly what to do. We made an emergency landing and I was taken to hospital where it was discovered that I had a brain tumour. It took a while to sink in. I was just 24. Even now, over two years later, some days I still find it hard to believe."
> Calum Wright

Some seizures aren't physical at all, and might only be observable to the patient themselves. You might experience *déjà vu*, feel like your mind is buffering, you might struggle to get language out (even though you know what you want to say), you might hear music or voices, or feel like your body is moving when it isn't.

All of these are also symptoms of stroke and epilepsy, so in any case are worth checking out. In brain tumours, seizures of one kind or another are believed to represent about half of all initial symptoms reported by patients that something might be wrong.

Headache

There are no pain receptors in the brain, which means your tumour and the brain around it cannot feel pain. However, when the tissues of the tumour, the brain, and any liquid build up (called odema) created by cell damage are struggling for space, the outward pressure around your skull can cause pain. That's because there are pain receptors in the membranes (meninges) *surrounding* the brain. Pressure on small cavities around the skull, in the sinuses, the back of the eyes and face can also create migraine like headaches.

> "One Sunday, my 23 year old son George was playing football with his uni friends. He had clashed heads with an opponent as he went to header a ball. He fell to the ground and was making strange utterances. He knew what was going on around him but could not speak. He was taken to Southampton General hospital, kept in overnight, monitored but not scanned. On the third day George was insistent that we went back to hospital. When we got out of the car I saw George clutching his head, and he was quite irritated but still I just imagined we

were only there to ease George's anxiety. After all here was a healthy 6ft 3 sportsman. The consultant commented that George seemed 'a bit flat for a 23 year old', and she ordered a CT scan. At first they thought George had had a stroke. Perhaps damage from the carotid artery due to the force of the football header incident. We were transferred to Charing Cross Hospital in London for further investigations and an MRI that night. A day or so later a consultant told me George had a lesion on the brain, and they drew the size of it. I was told it was a suspected tumour."
Jane Cooke, mother of George

Memory loss

The brain is responsible for short and long term memory, so pressure or abnormal activity in the memory areas are bound to send things awry. Brain tumour patients report forgetting names, numbers, place names and more, before their memory really begins to deteriorate and they perhaps forget faces, family, recent occurrences or even their own history. Once again, their closeness to stroke and dementia are not to be underestimated and are another key cause of misdiagnosis.

Speech and language difficulty

The frontal lobe, at the front of the brain, is a prime site for brain tumour growth. It is here that the brain cells responsible for speaking are located. It is not unusual for patients to experience a seizure where their ability to speak is affected. They may not be able to find the correct words for very familiar objects, or to pronounce even very simple words. Sometimes language might collapse completely, with the patient unable to put sentences together, producing mumbles, or words that appear all jumbled up. Most confusing of all, as I have experienced, is believing you are talking sense, when what is coming out of your mouth is completely confused and jumbled. Interestingly, this often temporary arrest in language ability can transfer to writing too. The patient may not be able to type or handwrite during a seizure like this.

> "I took my six year old son and his friend to a soft play area. The lady signing people in asked for my address then looked confused. The confusion was because I couldn't remember where we lived and my speech was slurred. After that everything was normal, and my wife laughed at me afterwards. A month later, I was working at home one evening when I came over very sick and ran to the toilet. I spent ages there feeling bad, but not vomiting. My wife came to check up on me after a while. I told her everything was okay, except this wasn't real language. She got me to sit down in the kitchen, and asked me questions. My complete lack of English scared her, and she called the emergency services."
> Graham Dunnett

Some brain tumour patients also report not being able to take in and process language. They can hear what is being said to them, but cannot make sense of the words as sentences, instructions or questions. This is more likely when the tumour is at the rear of the brain.

Mood change

This might be a temporary change, or something that grows over time. It is well documented that brain tumours can affect patients' temperaments. Those with brain tumours can become tetchy and short tempered. They may find themselves easily stressed by situations they'd previously found easy. They may react poorly to loud noises, or find it difficult to be in crowded places. I, for example, find it very difficult to be at a funfair with my children. There are too many lights, noises from all directions, movement everywhere you look, children running around and babies crying, even smells wafting around. I have to avoid getting into those situations if I want to stay in a good mood.

> "When she returned home mid June, after the biopsy, we went through the most difficult time. She was exhausted but also increasingly confused, distressed and at times belligerent. On several occasions she completely withdrew into herself and refused to talk. The person with whom I had never run out of conversation in 57 years – my identical twin sister, literally my other half – now had nothing to say to me. It was absolutely heartbreaking."
> Joanna Waters, sister of Sue Rossides

Hearing and sight loss

Testimonies of patients report a gradual narrowing of vision, or the ebbing away of hearing. These can both so easily be symptoms of other health conditions that it's unlikely a complaint of sight and hearing loss will have your doctor sending you to the MRI machine. However, linked to other symptoms such as imbalance, seizures and memory loss, doctors should at least consider some underlying neurological disorder, even if they don't suspect a brain tumour.

Specialist opticians are able to use their equipment to look through your eyes, and can detect if one of your optic discs are coming under pressure from behind. That may be an indication of a brain tumour or swelling at the front of the brain, and you're likely to be referred to hospital for a second opinion.

These are just a very few signs and symptoms of brain tumours, which you may or may not have noticed about yourself or a loved one. There are many others.

Unfortunately, there are also those who are later diagnosed with life limiting brain tumours who receive no warning at all. They might be having an MRI scan or a CAT scan for a completely different reason, perhaps a routine medical checkup, or after a sports injury, and only then is a tumour discovered in their brain.

Whichever way the tumour begins to show itself, the effects are no less devastating when they are revealed. While it may be a kind of relief to finally pin down why you have been feeling so dizzy, or sick, or finding it hard to cope with busy places, that's very quickly replaced with worry about the future.

Why symptoms?

What symptoms you experience will very much depend on where your tumour is located in the brain. No two brain tumours are the same size, nor in the same position, nor do they affect a particular patient in the same way. A larger size doesn't always mean a worse tumour. A certain location doesn't always spell better news. How you are affected can even depend on whether you are right or left handed.

It is true that only *you* can have *your* brain tumour. This is something to hold on to, because it means that other people's experience of what appears to be the same tumour might not necessarily be mirrored by your own.

Some people find hope in that fact, others will find it irrelevant. But it is worth noting that doctors, oncologists and neurologists are no more able to predict the future behaviour of your tumour – nor the impact it will have on you – than you are. They can detect patterns and make observations, but because every tumour and patient is different, they really must take every case as one of a kind. However, previous experience means they will often get your diagnosis right and know what to do about it, following generally accepted guidelines that have emerged from scientific data and practice.

In terms of symptoms, a few rules of thumb can fairly be applied. The location of the tumour is most likely to affect the functions of that particular part of the brain. But parts of the brain communicate with each other in a myriad of ways. The growing field of studying brain 'plasticity' is showing too that each of our brains are so different, having developed each individually according to our own early years, that there are no standardised areas that will always do the same things. Also, the control of many of our functions are actually spread all over our brains, rather than in one specific area. That means that brain tumours can have significant effects on brain functions that are nowhere near where the tumour is located.

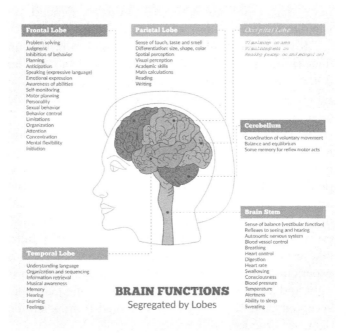

Frontal Lobe

Problem solving
Judgment
Inhibition of behavior
Planning
Anticipation
Speaking (expressive language)
Emotional expression
Awareness of abilities
Self-monitoring
Motor planning
Personality
Sexual behavior
Behavior control
Limitations
Organization
Attention
Concentration
Mental flexibility
Initiation

Parietal Lobe

Sense of touch, taste and smell
Differentiation: size, shape, color
Spatial perception
Visual perception
Academic skills
Math calculations
Reading
Writing

Occipital Lobe

Visualization on aims
Visualization on
Reading process on and inchings on?

Cerebellum

Coordination of voluntary movement
Balance and equilibrium
Some memory for reflex motor acts

Temporal Lobe

Understanding language
Organization and sequencing
Information retrieval
Musical awareness
Memory
Hearing
Learning
Feelings

Brain Stem

Sense of balance (vestibular function)
Reflexes to seeing and hearing
Autonomic nervous system
Blood vessel control
Breathing
Heart control
Digestion
Heart rate
Swallowing
Consciousness
Blood pressure
Temperature
Alertness
Ability to sleep
Sweating

BRAIN FUNCTIONS
Segregated by Lobes

But if you are able to obtain an MRI scan of your brain, you may be surprised and a little impressed – I certainly was – about how closely your symptoms are synonymous with the tumour's location.

My oligodendroglioma was around 4cm x 4cm x 6cm when it was first diagnosed, and was located in the middle and front of the left side of my head. It is a large tumour, deep in the left side of my brain and is so diffusely distributed throughout the brain and around blood vessels that it cannot be removed. It sits smack bang in the middle of the areas of my brain responsible for speech, motion and sensation. It stretches a little into memory and behaviour.

And my symptoms? Before medication, I experienced extreme language confusion, and sometimes still do. I would experience involuntary movement of my right limbs. During seizures I experience recurring memories of a childhood song, and I'm sorry to say my temper is occasionally far from what I'd like it to be. In short, I experienced symptoms that are spot on for the location of my brain tumour.

Mexico. James Campling was on holiday with his then girlfriend when he found he suddenly couldn't speak. Well, he could talk okay, but what he said wasn't coming out right. He could make noises. Half a word here, a garbled few syllables there. To him, James was making perfect sense, but his girlfriend just looked at him confused. She told him to stop messing around, and even James' reaction was to laugh about it.

Inside, though, he was scared. Nothing like that had ever happened to him and his immediate thought was that he was having a stroke. A few minutes later, though, his language cleared. Within 15 minutes he could talk again.

Then came Sudan. In his hotel having breakfast with a friend, James found he suddenly couldn't move. Or talk. He felt his head jerking to one side, but his friend detected nothing. She continued with her breakfast while James was undergoing what from inside felt like total mental collapse. She was later so unconvinced anything had happened, James thought he had not quite woken up yet and had dreamed it all.

It took a third seizure for him to take seriously what was happening to his body. And to his brain.

If you are going to have a serious epileptic seizure, there are probably few better places to have one than among dozens of medical professionals. James was attending an RAF nursing symposium when he began to go into a seizure. His fellow delegates immediately detected what was happening, and they sprang into action to make him safe while the seizure took place. Then they took him to an accident and emergency hospital department close to where the symposium was taking place.

He left there with a long list of specialist medics to see, and a list of appointments for tests. One of those tests was an MRI scan on his brain.

How are brain tumours diagnosed?

Once a doctor or a neurologist suspects you may have a brain tumour, or if they are not sure what is causing the symptoms you are having, you may be referred to have an MRI scan or a CT scan. Both of these take pictures inside your head, and will show up anything abnormal. An MRI scan is far more sensitive in imaging soft tissue and will show up tumours that are diffuse and of low intensity, compared with CT scans which offer a rougher picture.

In some countries, you can elect to have a brain scan simply by telling your doctor and medical insurance company that you want one. In other countries, such as the UK, which has a free-at-the-point-of-use health service (the NHS), a scan may be more difficult to obtain. That's because they are expensive and because brain tumours are relatively rare. Some doctors are reluctant to put you to the trouble, and the NHS to the cost, when your symptoms could more likely be related to stress, a temporary illness or something else.

It's hard to see their reasoning when your eventual scan does reveal a tumour. Indeed, the delay of diagnosis remains one of the most contentious issues in brain tumour detection and treatment. Suffice it to say, it's an ongoing discussion between charities, advocates and the medical establishment worldwide.

Computed Tomography

A computed tomography scan, known as a CT or CAT scan, is essentially a very high powered X-ray machine. It rotates around your head to produce a detailed 3D image of the tissues inside. If you've ever had an X-ray for a broken bone, the principle is the same. X-rays are projected from a machine, through your bones and tissues, and those that go through are 'imprinted' like a shadow onto sensors on the other side, creating an image. A CT scanner works the same way, except the machine rotates quickly, and the sensors on the other side rotate too, sending numerous images to a computer, allowing the build up of a 3D picture.

CT scans are good at examining bone breaks, because bones are hard and so are good at stopping X-rays from getting through to the sensors behind. Some advanced tumours are solid too, so show up well on a CT scan. But some brain tumours are more spread out into other brain tissue (known as diffuse), so don't stop X-rays so well. As such, they don't always show up on a CT scan. Astrocytomas can be very diffuse and CT scans are rarely used to monitor them once discovered.

Unlike the MRI scanner, the CT scanner doesn't enclose your whole body or head, so you shouldn't feel too claustrophobic having one. However, they do use high powered X-rays so aren't usually suitable for pregnant women. Otherwise, much of what you'll experience in a CT scan is the same as for an MRI which you're much more likely to have regularly.

> "After initially being taken to hospital for my seizures, they did some minor tests then asked me to come back in a few days time for more. I had a CT scan, and in the mid afternoon a registrar sat down with me and told me I might have a brain tumour. He said I would stay at hospital for three days. It was a totally strange three days: the first days of my having seizures and a brain tumour. To me, it just seemed pointless. If it was a tumour then someone would just cut it out and life would continue without any concerns. Life would be back to normal really soon."
> Graham Dunnett

Magnetic Resonance Imaging

If you have been diagnosed with a brain tumour, Magnetic Resonance Imaging (MRI) is something you will become extremely familiar with. Through a range of frequencies of magnetism and radio waves, the machine is able to take high resolution images of the inside of your brain, including soft tissue and liquid.

It builds up a slice by slice image of the whole of your brain; then computers put the slices together to create a 3D image of the brain and everything it contains. Your oncologist or brain surgeon will be able to 'scroll' through the slices, as well as examine a rotating 3D relief of your head. The MRI machine will take both scans that are just 12 slices at a time creating a very general picture, but also very detailed hundreds-of-slices images, the results of which are a wonder to behold.

Brain MRIs work by temporarily attracting the protons in hydrogen atoms contained in the water in your brain. In non-scientific language, the procedure makes the protons *point* in the same direction. When a radio wave is pulsed through the brain, the protons are temporarily released, before realigning again. Through measuring the energy they release on movement, the MRI scanner picks up the different rates at which those protons move. Those in different types of tissue move at different rates, creating the image.

For astrocytoma and glioblastoma tumours, you're very likely to be given a kind of dye during your MRI scan, through an injection. This contrasting agent, usually a chemical called gadolinium, enhances and improves the MRI image because it causes the protons in the brain tumour to move more quickly in response to the radio wave pulse. Especially in diffuse astrocytomas, the dye can show the extent of the tumour, where the brain tumour has infiltrated, its intensity and its size. It will also show the extent of blood vessel growth in the tumour. Together, these factors help make your brain tumour far more visible on MRI.

Gadolinium is generally regarded as very safe for most patients, though your doctor or radiology technologist will advise. Some will report a cold feeling in the arm when the dye is first administered. A very few patients may feel it makes them dizzy or sick. One in 1,000 may get a rash. One in 10,000 may suffer an allergic reaction.

If you are due to have a dye injected, your radiologists will ask about the function of your kidneys, as they will be responsible for ridding the body of the substance over the next 24 hours. They'll ask you other questions about allergies and pregnancy that may also be relevant. Usually, pregnant women will not be given an MRI or gadolinium in the early stages of pregnancy. Breast feeding can continue after a gadolinium injection.[8]

The end result of all this is that doctors will be able to take quite accurate measurements of a tumour's size, shape and level of diffusion. Medics are even able to make good estimations of the kind of brain tumour you have. All this without having to open up your head at all.

A diffuse anaplastic astrocytoma might appear on an MRI scan as a kind of thin cloud covering and infiltrating a single area of the brain. A glioblastoma may be a more solid lump, or it may be diffuse also. Within it might appear blank spaces where healthy brain cells have been killed off, and liquid is perhaps building up.

There is a growing field of neurology that specialises in being able to predict brain tumour type on image alone, though the accepted practice is still that an accurate diagnosis can only finally be achieved by taking a sample of the tumour and examining it under a microscope – called a biopsy.

Once you get used to seeing your own MRI scans, you'll be able to tell the difference between healthy tissue, brain tumour and areas of 'intensity' where the gadolinium is gathering, showing areas where the brain tumour is most active.

Whether you want to study your scans is personal

preference, but your doctor should give you copies if you request them and you can download free software from the internet that will allow you a closer look.[9]

Angiogenesis

Your doctors will use the MRI to look at how far the tumour is developing its own blood supply. Malignant tumours develop complex networks of blood vessels to support their own survival. This process is called angiogenesis.

One of the key signs that an initially low grade astrocytoma brain tumour has become malignant and invasive of the brain tissue around it is when it begins to tap into the brain's blood supply, and then goes on to create blood vessels of its own.

Some research has shown that angiogenesis is a key predictor of transformation from a Grade II astrocytoma to a Grade III. This means doctors may be able to treat your tumour as a Grade III, once it is clear angiogenesis is taking place, without having to carry out an additional biopsy.

Astrocytomas first acquire the blood which they need to function by co-opting the normal brain blood vessels, and growing along them. It is this that gives astrocytomas their invasive character, allowing them to spread like tentacles within the brain.

When the astrocytoma turns anaplastic, the cancer cells first starve the surrounding cells of blood, then they generate their own blood vessels. The end result is a steady blood flow and fuel for the cancerous brain cells, while the once healthy brain cells around them die off. A fully established brain tumour is like its own organ, with a self sustaining blood supply.

What happens during an MRI?

After any surgery, and during and after any other treatment you receive, it is very likely you will have regular MRI scans.

In the early stages after diagnosis and initial treatments, you're likely to be asked to have an MRI scan every three months – though this will vary according to your health centre. The regular scans allow your doctors to keep a close eye on the tumour and how treatment has affected it. They will quickly be able to see the gaps where the tumour has been removed by surgery, any scarring after radiotherapy, any remaining tumour, if the tumour is reducing in size, or if it is growing.

They'll use this information to judge whether to continue on three month monitoring, or if they can relax your schedule to six months or even longer. Some anaplastic astrocytoma and glioblastoma patients are on annual monitoring schedules, with only requests to inform their doctors if anything feels like it has changed. Perhaps a change in seizures, headaches or speech difficulties. (Obviously, this can be hard to judge for patients).

If you are a brain tumour patient, it's likely you will have had an MRI by now. But for friends and family, it is useful to briefly outline what will happen so they can help prepare you, and themselves.

The medical professional who operates your MRI machine is known as an MRI technologist, or a radiographer. Their job is to get you in and out of the machine safely, while ensuring they get the best images they can for your medical team. They'll be very happy to explain how it all works for you, though they won't be in the room when the actual MRI takes place. Though they are able to administer your contrast dye, through an intravenous injection, MRI technologists are not doctors or nurses.

They will not be able to show you your images, nor give you any indication of whether there have been any changes or if there is anything to worry about. They take the images, process them and then pass them on to a radiologist. This is a specialist doctor who can read and interpret the images.

In turn, the radiologist will pass their report to your oncologist or brain surgeon, who in turn will interpret and draw conclusions about your brain tumour. They may take the images to their own multidisciplinary team for advice or to bounce around ideas.

The first thing to remember about an MRI machine is that it is a massive magnet. You'll be asked three or four times whether you have any metal in or around your body. You'll need to fill in a form to testify you don't have a pacemaker, or shards of metal in your eyes, or metal joints, tattoos, contraceptive IUDs or otherwise anything else that might be attracted by a magnet. If you do have one of these things, your MRI technician will advise whether the procedure can go ahead. They may ask you to go into a CT scanner instead.

If you're due to have a contrast dye injection, you'll also be asked about the state of your kidneys and heart, particularly whether you've had any treatment or operations. That's because the MRI technician will want to ensure your organs will clear the dye from your body at a decent rate after it's been used in the imaging.

Be sure to tell your operator if you have claustrophobia, or if you're particularly nervous about enclosed spaces. They will help you with a sedative to help calm your fears if necessary.

You'll be asked to leave your keys, phone, belt and any other belongings in a locker. To save too much hassle in the MRI department, it's often best to attend in just a loose tracksuit, leaving jewellery and other bits at home. Note, though, that MRI rooms tend to be quite cold, so a T-shirt and shorts is probably not enough. You can choose whether to keep your shoes on or not, assuming they have no large pieces of metal in them.

If you're receiving a gadolinium dye, the MRI technician will take some non-enhanced images first, then give you the injection. They may simply come into the room in between scans, and give you the dye as an injection while you continue to lie still under the scanner, then leave the room to take more images.

More likely, they'll give you a cannula before you get onto the MRI bench. This is a very thin tube that is inserted into your veins, via a needle which is then removed. The cannula is then secured in place with a large, very sticky plaster. While you are lying in the MRI machine, they'll attach the cannula to a drip that contains the dye. They will then remotely begin the drip injection from their control room during the MRI scans.

The MRI machine itself is like a huge white doughnut. You'll lie down on a thin bench, and the technicians will either give you ear plugs or offer you headphones to block out some of the noise of the machine. Once you're lying down, they may put a cushion under your knees for your comfort, and they'll put sponges around your head to keep it still during the scans.

Remember, they'll be building up a picture of your brain slice by slice, so those slices need to line up. That means keeping your head in the same place over the five to ten minutes each scan takes.

Once the sponges are in place comes, arguably, the worst bit. You'll have a square plastic mask placed very closely over your head and face. Very often the mask has a mirror in it, so when you look up you can see your feet and usually the control room from where the MRI technicians will work during your scan. Finally, they'll give you a squeezable 'panic button' to use if you're feeling unwell or particularly uncomfortable during the scan.

After checking you're happy, you'll be gently rolled into the machine. The edges of the doughnut come very close to the plastic mask, and for those who don't like enclosed spaces it will take an act of will to calm your nerves at being so encased. I can't pretend to be scared of small spaces, but others say they have to take sedatives, or close their eyes for the whole time. Talk to your MRI technician before you go into the MRI room if you have concerns.

Once you're settled, the technicians will leave the room and the scans will begin. I've had dozens of scans, and still can't work out any pattern of what's going on.

There are very loud buzzes and bangs, whizzes and clicks. Scans vary from 30 seconds to around seven or eight minutes at a time. A few of them are so loud and intense, they seem to make the whole room around you shake.

Sometimes, if you're wearing headphones, the

MRI technicians will tell you how many scans are still to come, or how long the next one will be. They may play soft music, or even music you choose if you're lucky, but you can't get away from it being a very loud affair.

And because you're having to keep very still and keep looking in the same direction, a pretty boring one. The key is to try to relax from the get-go, allowing your arms and legs to flop and to release tension from your back. It'll be much more comfortable to maintain a relaxed rather than tense position for 45 minutes.

Once the scan is over, your MRI technician will return to the room, roll you out of the doughnut, and help you to your feet. You'll (rather painfully in my experience) have the sticky plaster and the cannula removed, and you'll be sent on your way.

It will be very rare to get any kind of results from your MRI scan soon after the scan itself. Unless you are already on a hospital ward, you may be asked to come back for your results with your brain surgeon or oncologist days, weeks or even a number of weeks later. These are nervous days but radiologists and other medical professionals need time to process all the images, and they will often consult with colleagues, known as your multidisciplinary team (MDT), about the scans, before they decide on what to advise you to do next.

Despite what some would have you believe, MRI scans are extremely safe. They cannot affect your brain or brain tumour, and the contrast dye contains chemicals that encourage your body to process it quickly and eject it from the body through your urine, without affecting your health.

Results day

In brain tumours, every doctor's appointment, every scan and every meeting with your consultant feels like 'results day'. Every new appointment could be the one you're told the latest bad news, that your current situation has changed, or that you need new treatment.

My wife and I pretend to ourselves that we've got used to doctors' appointments, but in reality we can both feel the tension between us as an MRI result approaches. We don't know what to expect, and we try not to pick apart what might happen, but it is difficult.

What I have discovered is that working with my wife to write down some very specific questions for my oncologist or consultant has helped enormously, in the run up to results day. In their office, it's easy to forget the vital questions you want to ask and to end up not getting the information you want. I write a series of questions, and we vow not to leave the office until we get them answered, or understand that they don't apply.

Most of the time, the questions centre around whether there has been growth (or shrinkage) in the tumour, and what that indicates about how the treatment is working. I'll report any new or ongoing symptoms, and ask about their significance. I'll then ask what happens next. Because I am particularly interested in the detail, I'll ask for print outs of the radiologist's report about my latest MRI scan. When there is something significant happening, I'll ask for the scans themselves. In my current hospital, it means going through a bureaucratic process under UK legislation to formally ask for my medical records. Other hospitals I've been cared for in have simply handed me a CD of my images before I've left.

> "George got used to the MRI process pretty quickly, but that is not to say he liked it. He endured it. He hated the smell of the hospital, he disliked going through the doors. The uncertainty, the anxiety that would build. That sick feeling in the pit of the stomach never left and always increased a thousandfold as George's name was called to see the consultant. I cannot understand why there was a minimum of two weeks' wait from MRI to results. That wait was arduous. After George's final admission to hospital in December 2015, the one thing he was relieved about was no more scans and no more hospital visits."
> Jane Cooke, mother of George

A report that your tumour is stable should be taken as a great sign, and something to cling to. But if the news is bad, it is important that you try not to close down and exit the consultant's clinic at the earliest opportunity. This is your opportunity to take your time, get as much information as possible, and talk to the experts in front of you about next steps.

In the UK, brain tumour patients are often allocated a clinical nurse specialist (CNS) – a medical professional who supports the oncologist, and can provide you with extra information and support if the oncologist is too busy to devote enough time to you. They are likely to be your key contact. In most cases, you're perfectly entitled to ask for a break and then see either your oncologist or your CNS before you leave. They'll give you a chance to ask any questions that have occurred to you back in the waiting room.

I almost always seem to come out of my meetings with more questions than answers, and often feel frustrated that I can't get back to my oncologist with my supplementary questions once I've had a chance to discuss the meeting with my wife and brother. Your ability to pose these extra questions will depend on your medical team, but there should at least be your CNS or equivalent to approach in the clinical centre which is responsible for your care to pose any additional questions. If not, brain tumour charities may help you with the information you're seeking, or even advocate on your behalf with the hospital or clinician.

For Duncan Weaver, waiting for results day after each of his three month scans was always agony. But it was the first scan after initial diagnosis that was the worst. Duncan and Loes just didn't know what to expect, and feared that the scan would already show growth in his low grade tumour.

That first scan showed no change and was a massive relief. The consultant hadn't beaten about the bush, but told the couple as soon as they walked in that the tumour was stable. They were shown the first MRI scan and the latest scan side by side, and the consultant explained what to expect if the tumour began to transform.

Seeing the scans up close helped the methodical and logical Duncan to translate what his consultant was saying into reality. It made it easer to process the information.

For more than a year and a half, those results meetings never gave any indication of tumour change.

But results day never got any easier. Duncan and Loes would get tetchy with each other. They didn't speak much about the 'maybes', perhaps not wanting to voice their fears, but only about the logistics of getting to the hospital on time. As the meeting approached, Duncan's symptoms seemed to become worse: as if his body was preparing him for what he would be told.

Duncan and his wife did what many of us with brain tumours do. They lived from MRI to MRI, allowing the next test to rule their life. 'Let's wait until we have the results of the next scan,' 'We'd better wait for the next result before we book a holiday.'

Only after more than a year of life in three month chunks did the couple realise they had to take control, before the MRIs took control of them. From that moment they would look ahead. They would live like Duncan had not been diagnosed. They would plan holidays. They finally bought a house. Most significantly of all, they decided to try for a baby.

Transforming from low to high grade

> "It was explained that George's lesion was suspected to be an astrocytoma of low grade. It was very large but operable. We were told it was the best of tumours to have in the best of places, the left frontal lobe. In fact, they were so confident they offered watch and wait, or surgery. But George said he wanted surgery and as soon as possible, and I could sense he was confident in his decision."
> Jane Cooke, mother of George

I was diagnosed with a Grade II oligodendroglioma. It

was a low grade tumour that I understood was bound to transform one day into a more malignant anaplastic tumour. At the time I wrote my first brain tumour book, *Brain Tumours: Living Low Grade*, it was about living with an ultimately life limiting, but currently stable disease.

As part of that book, I interviewed dozens of patients with the same tumour as mine, as well as patients with low grade astrocytomas. We all knew that one day our tumours would most probably transform into higher grade tumours.

We were all engaged in living in three or six month chunks, waiting for MRI scans to give us the latest update. The general attitude was that though we were experiencing symptoms and serious life limitations because of our tumours, many of us were generally healthy and living relatively normal lives. Even though those lives had all been changed beyond recognition.

Since I wrote that book, my tumour has transformed into a higher grade: an anaplastic oligodendroglioma. I have had to have intensive cancer treatment to halt its growth and impact. One of the worst parts was telling friends and family that I needed to start treatment. They were puzzled about why this was suddenly happening. I was still very healthy, nothing had changed in my behaviour, ability or fitness.

In their minds – and this is a notion shared by many brain tumour patients who have contributed to these pages – the tumour had somehow gone away. I wasn't dying, so I was as good as cured. When I was first diagnosed, there was much wailing and love and visits and gifts and donations, yet I was super well. Now, as I got underway with treatment, it was greeted by little more than a puzzled shrug from all but those who properly understood how my tumour works.

A combination of symptoms indicated to me that things may have begun to transform. My epileptic seizure activity, previously relatively well controlled, went awry. I was having up to 30 localised, partial seizures every day, where previously I'd only have one or two. I'd have a constant metallic taste in my mouth, and felt far more fatigued than I had been.

I wasn't surprised to learn that the surgeon declared there was almost certainly intensification in the tumour in certain areas. Apart from the wearing down of nearly a year of treatment since then, transition does not yet feel as if it has had a significant impact on my life. I don't particularly feel more scared than before. My doctor has told me I am doing well. The oligodendroglioma is a cousin of the astrocytoma, but behaves quite differently even when it has transformed.

Astrocytoma patients have had various responses to the transformation of their tumours. Some have taken it more or less in their stride: another step in the journey. We expected the worst each MRI, and were surprised that the worst hadn't happened until now.

For others, though, transformation came as a total shock. Some did not understand the implications of it, others were – through no fault of their own – unprepared.

> "Two years after my first seizure at the play
> centre with my son, I had the usual MRI scan.
> Results day was soon afterwards and that
> afternoon I was told my tumour had changed
> greatly and surgery was needed. It felt

somewhat horrific. We thought I had years not months. We crumbled from this news. In the weeks waiting for the surgery my health declined rapidly and speech, writing and walking was all a struggle. The surgery was our only hope. We were both anxious and fearful of the unknown."
Graham Dunnett

Diagnosis

WHEN JAMES CAMPLING made that phone call from the train between Finland and Norway, he had an inkling about what his doctor was calling about. The dozen missed calls indicated a desperation that couldn't be ignored.

The three seizures he'd had – in Mexico, Sudan and at the RAF nursing conference before he'd left for Scandinavia – had convinced him and his doctor that, at the very least, he had epilepsy. His inability to speak and inability to move during a seizure were proof positive of that. But James knew more. The internet is generous in that way.

James knew that around half of people who experience partial focal seizures like the ones he'd experienced were later diagnosed with a brain tumour.

As the doctor was speaking down the crackly overseas line through the Finnish wilderness, James was initially shocked and nearly broke down. The MRI had shown a mass on his brain that was almost certainly a brain tumour. It would need a biopsy at least, probably brain surgery to remove it.

But within minutes James had gathered himself together. Wasn't that what RAF corporals were supposed to do? He put together a plan to get home. At the next station, James leapt from the train ready to head to the nearest airport. He should have stayed on the train because he seemed to have disembarked at the most remote station in Finland.

But he eventually ended up in Helsinki waiting for a flight the next day. That evening was probably the loneliest of his life, despite spending so much time alone as a hobbyist solo explorer. He went down to the near to empty bar in the Holiday Inn, propped himself against it and bought the person next to him a pint.

The guy got the full story.

The typical journey

What's going to happen now? That's the first question that will have crossed your mind if you have been diagnosed with an anaplastic astrocytoma or a glioblastoma. It is very likely you have already, or are about to experience, the first steps in what you may begin referring to as 'your journey' for the lack of any better way of putting it.

Every patient is different, and every brain tumour is different, but there are some broad brush steps that might be typical for a patient. It might be that your journey looks nothing like the following, but this is the shape recommended and followed by most brain tumour oncologists worldwide.

This book goes into much more detail about each of these areas, but this quick guide may answer your immediate questions.

Image based diagnosis

Following a seizure, blackout, stroke like episode or headaches, you may be given a series of tests. These will probably include an MRI scan, which will identify whether you have some kind of brain tumour. Your surgeon, neurologist or oncologist will be able to tell you with some certainty what kind of brain tumour type it is just by looking at the scan. They won't be able to tell its specific genetic makeup, and are very unlikely to be able to tell you how serious it is.

Surgery

If your oncologist thinks you may have an anaplastic astrocytoma or a glioblastoma, it's likely they will want to remove as much of it as they can. Indeed, this is now the accepted practice for all but the most benign types of tumour. This is called 'debulking', or 'partial resection'. The more tumour they can get out, the better. But they will not operate on areas of the tumour that are very close to or intermeshed with the parts of your brain responsible for principal functions like movement, speech, memory or thinking.

Your surgery will either be under general anaesthetic (you'll be totally unconscious), or it'll be an awake craniotomy where you'll be woken up part of the way through. The latter is so you can respond to questions and carry out simple movements, so the surgeon can match the parts of your brain they are working on with the parts of your brain responsible for movement, memory and speech.

Biopsy

If you have debulking surgery, a piece of the

tumour will be sent for testing. If your surgeon has concluded your tumour is too dangerous to operate on at all – say because it has blood vessels running through it, or it is located in the middle of the movement areas of your brain – then they will most likely just carry out a needle biopsy.

Under general or local anaesthetic, a hole will be drilled in your skull. If the tumour is close to the surface, they will use a hollow needle to extract a piece of tumour. If it is deeper, they will carry out a stereotactic biopsy. This is a needle again, but guided by computer, MRI and CT scans, to ensure a sample of the 'worst' parts of the tumour are taken. A number of samples will be taken.

Histological diagnosis

After your biopsy or surgery, the brain tumour tissue will be sent for analysis. Experts will examine the tissue under a microscope and use dyes to create a full picture of your tumour. It is only after the biopsy that you will be given the tumour's 'histology', the definition of the tumour based on its difference from normal cell shape and behaviour.

In short, you will be told what kind of brain tumour you have. Unless you ask for it, the histology you are given is likely to be relatively broad brush: for example, an anaplastic astrocytoma or a glioblastoma. There are actually many subsets of these tumours, but their names and definitions might not mean too much to you at this stage.

Your biopsy will also have enabled a view of the genetic markers of your brain tumour. This looks at the DNA in the cells of your tumour, to investigate whether particular genes have been corrupted, changed, have disappeared or have been paired incorrectly. Genetic signatures are extremely important in all cancers, and this is discussed in detail later.

Treatment

After your biopsy, your multidisciplinary team will consider again how the information they've gained will affect how they would like to treat you. First for those who've not yet had surgery will be the question of whether surgery might now be appropriate. Second will be the question of what chemotherapy and radiotherapy you should have.

If your team discover that you have a low grade astrocytoma, rather than an anaplastic one, they may decide it is best to monitor your tumour and do nothing more for the time being. This is called 'watch and wait', and you will be monitored by MRI every three months or so.

If your team concludes you have an anaplastic astrocytoma or glioblastoma, they'll almost certainly recommend you begin radiotherapy or chemotherapy. Most likely, they'll recommend both at the same time as for most breeds of these types of tumour this is proven to be the most effective approach because it attempts to rid the brain of any cancer cells remaining after surgery.

Radiotherapy

You're likely to begin radiotherapy almost as soon as any surgery scars have healed. The standard is to have six weeks of five-days-a-week radiotherapy, but your treatment will be designed around your needs. Each session lasts about 15 minutes, but it really can wear down your motivation and your energy levels.

There are a number of types of radiotherapy. Your oncologist will advise you what they are, and why they recommend a particular type for you.

Chemotherapy

Most likely, you'll be placed on a drug called temozolomide (the brand name is Temodal, or Temodar in the United States). This you'll take for anything between three to six cycles, perhaps more. You're likely to take it alongside radiotherapy, as it makes radiotherapy work better. Like all chemotherapy, it's toxic. That means it kills cancer cells, but will make you feel pretty rubbish too. Some patients find they can't tolerate the drug at all. You will almost certainly experience some side effects. Throughout chemotherapy and radiotherapy, your oncologist will monitor you and your side effects, and will MRI you to see how well the treatment is working.

After treatment

This is where patients' experiences are most likely to begin to differ. For some, treatment will have done a very good job at knocking the tumour back, and some are put on a three month watch and wait protocol. For others, tumours grow back very quickly and further action needs to be taken. That might be more surgery, more chemotherapy (perhaps of a different kind), immunotherapy (a specific kind of chemotherapy that is still developing), or enrolment on a clinical trial of some kind.

In worst case scenarios, doctors may recommend a treatment or a care plan that will attempt to maintain quality of life for as long as possible, but which unfortunately has no prospect of affecting the disease.

After two years of being turned away by doctors, it would be a standin medic that would change Lian Davis and her mother Gillian's life forever.

Gillian's family doctor was away, so she saw a locum about her reoccurring headaches, and the sensitivity of even having her hair brushed. The doctor wasted no time. Lian was to take Gillian to hospital immediately. There an emergency MRI scan would be organised. A brain scan? Lian was more puzzled than ever. It was from one extreme to another; a few paracetamol to a full on brain scan.

The waiting room at the hospital didn't help. Lian and her mother were surrounded by people who were obviously seriously ill. She tried not to look, but couldn't help feeling sorry for the other patients waiting for scans: the sides of their heads sported huge scars, or were covered in bandages. At least something was being done about the headaches, Lian thought. She didn't utter to her mother the growing and terrifying thoughts forming in her mind.

Gillian wasn't good with confined spaces, but the radiologists gave her some sedatives to calm her nerves before she was fed into the MRI machine. Twenty minutes later, she was out of the machine and on her way home. A consultant would get back to her in a week or so. The doctor called the next day. Gillian was to come back to hospital. That's when Lian's stomach dropped through the floor. She knew what was coming. Her mother had a huge mass on the brain. It needed to be operated on immediately.

And by immediately, he meant that day: an emergency biopsy would see if the mass was a brain tumour. And if it was, what type of brain tumour it was. Lian, her sister and brother fell apart. But their strong, calm mother told them it would be okay.

"Really Mom?" asked Lian, realising she'd always looked to her kind mother for the answers to her own and the world's problems.

"Yes, it will," Gillian had said.

Gillian proceeded into theatre. Lian could think of nothing but escape. She headed for the car park and sat there in the car crying, every new Google result she brought up on her phone conjuring up worse and worse scenarios.

In the space of a few hours, Lian learned about low and high grade brain tumours, about malign and benign cancers, about the possibility of treatment and cure. Surely her kind, wonderful mother wouldn't be one of the 50 percent of patients whose brain lesion was malignant? Surely it couldn't be cancer? Surely she would be cured? Too many people wouldn't be able to cope without her.

What made her most angry was that simply typing in her mother's most basic symptoms over the last two years pointed so obviously towards a brain tumour. Why hadn't Lian done that search before? More importantly, how could their family doctor have missed something so obvious?

When Gillian came out of surgery for her biopsy, Lian and her siblings tried to hide their surprise. They were delighted that their mother gave them a thumbs up as soon as she saw them, but none of them could help but notice Gillian's long black hair. It had been shaved from the whole of one side of her head.

But at least she was alive, sitting up and making an effort to show she was okay and in good spirits. She knew how desperately concerned her kids would be.

The difficulty of diagnosis

Stories abound about adults with brain tumours failing to get a proper diagnosis, despite going back to doctors a number of times with headaches, dizzy spells, seizures, and other key symptoms of brain tumours.

It's no exaggeration to describe patients as angry that they have had to return to their family doctors, specialists and others time and again, only to be sent away as if they were wasting time. Growing pains, puberty, migraines, stress, poor diet and malingering have all been levelled at patients who, it later turns out, have brain tumours.

Some, and these are the angriest of patients and families, have been turned away again and again by medics, only to be admitted in an emergency days or weeks later. Then they're immediately diagnosed with a brain tumour and find themselves in surgery within 24 hours.

Brain tumour charities and pressure groups make much of these stories. My own correspondents illustrate this understandable frustration too. But at the risk of playing devil's advocate, it is perhaps worth registering a note of caution when laying blame at a local doctor or medical centre's door for not spotting a brain tumour.

Brain tumours quickly become the very centre of our own and our families' worlds after we become diagnosed. But it is important to remember that they are actually very rare, and that many local or family doctors may encounter only two or three cases in their whole career. At the same time, they may encounter countless cases of stress, migraine, epilepsy and so on.

How often did you encounter brain tumours before you experienced a diagnosis in your family? I suspect only among friends of friends, or via the television.

When presented with a patient who reports dizziness or severe headaches, it's simply a fact that the symptoms are more likely to be down to migraine or another cause than a brain tumour. Our doctors will act according to their knowledge and experience, and the likelihood of one particular condition over another. Doctors simply don't have the resources to send every patient with a reoccurring headache for an expensive scan in a hospital.

It is also worth saying that doctors do spot brain tumours, and they do refer people with brain tumour symptoms to specialists. But because these aren't regarded as failures, their pre-diagnosis actions aren't highlighted.

My own diagnosis ran pretty much to this structure, with my family doctor referring me to a stroke clinic after my seizures, who then ran a number of tests including an MRI scan. But even my stroke consultant didn't suspect a brain tumour when I first saw him.

Without an MRI or CT scan, diagnosing a brain tumour is very difficult. Because the cancer occurs in the brain, it can cause any number of symptoms that can so easily be mistaken as a different problem: and in fact, are more likely to be. From bowel problems to hearing difficulties, imbalance to language confusion, there are any number of symptoms that our doctors have to deal with where brain tumours might be furthest from their mind.

And when doctors fail to communicate well with each other, each spotting different symptoms but not joining the dots, that can lead to the medical establishment failing to see the bigger picture they've created.

Of course, there are cases of real misdiagnosis, negligence and poor patient care. I do not wish to denigrate these cases, but only to strike some balance when patients and loved ones are looking for someone, anyone, to blame.

Treatment

THOUGH IT CAN sometimes feel like you're in this alone, you will accumulate a team of medical experts and others who will one way or another become involved in your life. Their titles and roles may be confusing, and medics aren't always forthcoming about what they're supposed to be doing to, or for, you at any time.

Though you might only see one consultant on a regular basis, perhaps a particular surgeon or a neurologist, there will actually be a whole team of doctors, radiologists, nurses and oncologists looking after your case.

Behind the scenes, this team will be discussing your brain tumour, discussing your treatment, and making recommendations about what should happen next. It wasn't until I saw a television programme about brain tumours and a section where about a dozen people, including some junior and trainee doctors, were sitting in a lecture theatre looking at someone's MRI scans, that I understood properly the role of the multidisciplinary team (known as the MDT).

Most effective brain tumour centres put an MDT at the heart of their work with patients. That's pretty reassuring. It is worth highlighting the key figures you are likely to encounter, some of whom will be key players in your MDT.

Family doctor (GP or MD)

It was probably your local or family doctor to whom you first reported any problems, unless your tumour was found as an accident or in an emergency. Day to day, you may only see your GP to get drugs prescriptions and sick letters signed, perhaps for the occasional check up and to help deal with side effects of the tumour or its treatment. GPs are generally copied into all the major letters and emails various consultants send to each other. In an ideal world, they'll know what's going on with your tumour at any one time. But they often don't, and you'll probably keep them more up to date than your specialists will.

Neurologist

This brain doctor will most likely be a specialist in brain tumours, and possibly epilepsy too, but they're unlikely to be a surgeon. They will follow your MRI scans and advise you about growth, the effectiveness of treatment and possibly be responsible for your anti-seizure medication.

Oncologist

This is a cancer doctor, an expert in the disease and its treatment. They're usually specialists in a particular field too, so you can expect yours to be a brain cancer oncologist (neuro oncologist), though they may specialise in other cancers also. They'll advise on non-surgical treatments, such as radiotherapy and chemotherapy, guide you through the regimes, monitor results and make changes accordingly. They'll also write prescriptions for nausea drugs (called antiemetics), steroids, and any other medicines.

Surgeon/neurosurgeon

Though you may not meet a brain surgeon unless you need to have a biopsy or surgery to reduce the size of your tumour, they're likely to be part of your MDT. Ahead of surgery, you're likely to discuss with them what operation they'd like to do, how they'll go about it, and of course they and their team will be the ones getting inside your skull on the day. Depending on how you respond to surgery, you may or may not see a brain surgeon regularly.

Neuropathologist

A neuropathologist diagnoses diseases of the central nervous system by looking at a sample of brain tissue under a microscope. They establish the type and grade of your tumour, and carry out tests to determine its genetic makeup. They are the ones who will write up your histology – the cellular diagnosis of your cancer – though you may never meet them.

Registrar/junior doctor

A registrar is a qualified doctor who is studying and specialising in a particular aspect of medicine over five to ten years. They'll be training under a very experienced consultant (surgeon, oncologist, neurologist). They see patients alongside the consultant, or sometimes in place of them.

Clinical nurse specialist (CNS)

Most brain cancer doctors and many neurologists should have a CNS working directly with them in the UK; there are equivalents in other countries. They take much of the pastoral, support and some administrative work out of the consultant's hands, and are likely to be in more regular contact with you. It's them you're likely to first approach if your symptoms change, or if you're worried about an aspect of your treatment.

Most are experts in brain tumours, and are likely to have seen much of what you're experiencing before. They will make referrals to other services such as counselling or physiotherapy if you need them.

Radiologists

Doctors who use images to diagnose and treat disease. Radiologists use your MRI images to diagnose, treat and manage medical conditions. They will plan your radiotherapy. They will write a report for the neurologist, oncologist or surgeon, which along with the images, blood counts and other results will help your MDT to determine their next move.

Radiographers

These come in two types, diagnostic and therapeutic. They are not doctors. The basic difference is that a diagnostic radiographer will oversee imaging like MRIs, while a therapeutic radiographer administers radiotherapy treatment.

They may have a good knowledge about brain tumours, but neither are likely to supply information directly to patients.

You and your family

While it can sometimes feel like your medical care is out of your control, it really isn't. Except in very special circumstances, doctors and surgeons can't make us undergo any intervention without our consent. What's often missing is that the patient doesn't properly understand what's being offered to them and so offers their consent blindly. It is important you feel part of your MDT. Sometimes you'll have to push your doctors or your CNS, if you have one, to be taken seriously and consulted for your opinions and questions.

Getting a second opinion

Medicine can sometimes feel like a lottery, particularly in public health systems like the NHS in the UK. There are very real disparities between health quality in general, and responses to particular medical conditions, depending on where the patient lives. If you are not paying for your care, either directly or through a health insurance scheme, it is likely the medical care you receive will simply be what you end up with rather than something you choose.

This may be no bad thing. Cancer, brain tumours, brain surgery and oncology are well developed fields, and effective protocols are increasingly shared worldwide to ensure you get the appropriate treatment for the kind of brain tumour that you have.

But what about if you are not sure about the medical opinion you have received, or you actively doubt an opinion? While in the UK the NHS does not give us a right to a second opinion, most doctors will not feel offended or prevent you from seeking one.

Their primary interest is in your health. Whether a second doctor confirms or contradicts your main doctor's opinion is good for both doctors, and for you. It will double check your doctor's work, and force them to look again at the evidence in the face of an alternative opinion. Ultimately, it will be up to you whose advice you take.

In the NHS, you are likely to be able to get another doctor's opinion in the field of brain tumours for free. Additionally, or alternatively, you may wish to attempt to get a private sector opinion. Note, though, many private medical consultants also work in the public sector. There's no evidence that medical treatment or opinions are better simply because you are paying for them.

In countries where there is a medical insurance system, it is more likely to be up to your insurance company whether you will be able to seek a second opinion. Here, though, the pressure of competition and media can play a part. Will insurance companies really prevent their patients from seeking clarity, when the consequences of your first doctor getting it wrong might be extremely damaging to the insurer's reputation? You are advised to seek permission from your insurer before seeking another opinion, otherwise you may risk not being covered for the consultation.

Note that seeking extra opinions will always add time to your brain cancer journey, which may or may not be relevant to your particular circumstances.

Lian's mum Gillian rested in hospital following her biopsy, the whole family already resigned to the fact she would need a bigger operation to remove the lesion in her brain – whatever the biopsy revealed.

At 36, Lian was the eldest of her siblings. On a hospital visit, Gillian drew her daughter close to the bed to speak to her in private. Lian's mother asked her to hide the results of the biopsy from her, and to be the doctor's main point of contact from now on. It was an enormous weight to lay on her shoulders.

Lian looked towards her mother's partner, but he shrugged and said he couldn't take it. Lian screamed inside. She didn't want the responsibility either. She didn't want to know; she didn't want to be the one to tell others that their wonderful mother might die. She didn't want to have to hide the truth from her mum either.

But Lian came to a realisation. For the time being, Gillian couldn't head up the family and be everyone's rock as she had been. Though she resented Gillian's partner for it, Lian knew she would have to take over.

Results day came around all too quickly, especially now she would have to be the one processing all the information for the rest of the family.

As the consultant entered the room, there was no delay. For Lian, his approach was too matter of fact.

"It's not good news," the doctor said.

Gillian's partner stood and walked out of the office, just like that. He left the doctor to explain to Lian alone that her mother had a glioblastoma. Lian was familiar with the word, but there were so many types of brain tumour it was hard to remember them all. It was then he told her that her mother's brain tumour was a Grade IV.

Lian knew what that meant.

The tears came and she was desperate to stay in the office, waiting for the doctor to change his mind. Eventually, she found the strength to leave. How could she tell her family and what was she going to tell her mum?

With her siblings, she didn't need to. The puffy face and avoiding their eye contact told the whole story. At Gillian's bedside, Lian told her mother she needed to have a major operation, but that some of the tumour might have to be left behind. There was a lot that could be done to stop the tumour returning. They'd need hope and determination, she told her: "It's not going to get you, Mom. Let's do this together."

"It's bad, isn't it?" Gillian said quietly.

Lian closed her eyes, trying in vain to prevent the tears returning. She held her mum's hand and nodded gently.

Surgery is the front line of defence against glioblastoma and anaplastic astrocytoma brain tumours. If they can get to it, your surgeon will want to take out as much of the tumour as possible. And usually as soon as possible.

The more tumour a surgeon is able to remove, the better the patient's chances of a longer progression free life (the time when the tumour is not growing), and the longer their ultimate life expectancy.

Brain surgeons are experts in their trade and will often operate on two or three patients in a day, depending on their case load. The medical recovery period from brain surgery is likely to be the same as from any other type of operation under anaesthesia, though it should be noted that brain surgery can leave short and long term effects on a patient's mobility and ability to understand (cognition).

Peter Black, an experienced north American brain surgeon and author of *Living With a Brain Tumour,* estimates a 92 to 95 percent chance that brain surgery will go smoothly, with complications in only five to eight percent of cases.[10] And as his book was written more than 10 years ago, there's every reason to suspect surgery has now become even more successful.

The process of brain surgery

Over the following paragraphs, I describe in detail the rather icky process of brain surgery. It's not a bloody procedure, but you may find it difficult to read if you or a loved one are about to undergo surgery.

Your brain surgery will be based on very accurate MRI scans taken of your head, in the run up to and on the day of surgery itself. During the surgery, your surgeon may use real time CT scans and other imaging to guide their hand, as well as computer guided instruments.

Surgery takes place under a very experienced brain surgeon, who will have the very latest equipment at their disposal to ensure the surgery is as safe and effective as it can be. This could include MRI tractographs (a kind of photograph), functional MRI (real time imaging of your brain), and computer guidance based on your brain scans. Even lasers are used to zap brain cells, in some circumstances.

Before you begin surgery, you may have circular stickers stuck on your face, temples, neck and head. They may need to shave some of your hair either before you go under anaesthetic, or while you are under.

The stickers will be used as a guide, helping to keep your head in exactly the right place during surgery. Beams of light will be lined up with the stickers while you are on the surgery bench. Also, a metal frame may be attached to your head, with pins screwed into your skull from either side. Don't worry, you'll be given a local or general anaesthetic before this takes place. Suitably 'framed' and held still, your skull will be presented to your surgeon. This framing allows the surgeon to use computer guided imagery to get right to the tumour. It may not be necessary if your tumour is on the surface of the brain, or easy to access.

The surgical team will make an incision in your skin, peeling back enough to get a good opening to your brain. They will then use a surgical saw to create a hole in your skull bone called a bone flap. This will either be moved aside, or removed completely, providing access to your brain. It is through this hole that the surgeon will cut into your brain, or cut away parts, in order to get to the tumour.

First they will be seeking to get a sample of tumour, which may be tested immediately to see what type of tumour you have. Second, your surgeon will try to remove as much of the tumour as possible. It is at this point that you might be woken up, if you are having an awake craniotomy (see below).

When the surgeon has done as much as they can, they might insert some chemotherapy wafers – coin sized discs of chemotherapy drug in solid form – close to the site of the tumour. If you have oedema (liquid swelling on the brain) they may insert a drainage tube, to allow excess liquid to leak away after the operation. The surgeon will then close up the brain and the surrounding tissues using stitches that will dissolve over time. They'll then replace the bone flap, securing it with pins, and then roll back the skin over your head and stitch it together.

Very often the result is a long, clean, curved scar across the side of the head. You may also find you have stitches in each side of your head, where the pins from a metal frame were screwed in. Surgeons, their staff, nurses and your aftercare team will go to great lengths to protect this scar tissue. This is to keep it neat, but also to prevent infection of the scar. You'll be advised how to care for it. If it does get infected, you may be given antibiotics.

In the early weeks it will look brutal, as if a pirate has attempted to take off your head with a cutlass. Once you have had the stitches removed – often at your local medical centre – you will hopefully see the swelling retreat and the hair return. Some of us get away with barely visible scars, others are able to use new hairstyles or wigs to hide them should they want to.

Awake craniotomy

"I had an awake craniotomy. This lasted five hours with two hours awake and a speech therapist asking me relevant questions as the operation continued. I came out of the surgery chatting non stop and back to my old self. It was a miracle. Within the first hour I was having a roast dinner. When I got home life quickly got back to pre-tumour days. Within three weeks I was holidaying with friends on the south coast. The surgery gave me my life back."
Graham Dunnett

A very common form of surgery for a glioblastoma and anaplastic astrocytoma is an awake craniotomy. It's used when the tumour is close to parts of your brain responsible for movement, speech, language and memory. For the majority of the surgery, sometimes lasting eight hours or more, you will be under anaesthetic, unconscious and unaware of what the surgical team are doing inside your brain.

But for some periods during the surgery, you will be awoken by a reduction of the amount of anaesthetic you are under. Strong painkillers prevent you from feeling any pain during this time.

With you awake, the surgical team will talk to you while the surgeon prods part of your brain. As you are asked questions, urged to talk about your holidays, or requested to do certain tasks such as squeeze a nurse's hand, the surgeon is able to 'map' the parts of your brain which are responsible for functions such as movement, speech and cognition.

Once it is clear that prodding a certain part of brain tissue makes your speech become garbled, for example, the surgeon will mark it so that they can avoid any cutting in that area. Slowly, with lots of hard work by you and your surgical team, a picture is built up of where the surgeon can intervene. It is really only then that a surgeon will understand how much of the tumour they will be able to take out, without damaging your functionality. You will then be put back under anaesthetic while the majority of debulking takes place.

After surgery, when you wake, your doctors will test your speech, movement and reactions again, in the hope that the whole operation has had minimal impact on your brain function.

Though it sounds challenging, awake craniotomies

are regarded as safe, and have led to a giant leap forward in terms of the amount of tumour surgeons have been able to take out. Where previously overcautious, they've been able to cut further into brain tissues, helping to extend the lives of brain tumour patients without causing further damage. For reassurance and intrigue, you may be interested to see an awake craniotomy on YouTube which will give you a very clear idea of what to expect.

> "I had an awake craniotomy resection of the tumour. I can vaguely recall the operation. I know the woman who checked my capabilities prior the op was kind enough to sit with me during it. She talked to me when the surgeons wanted to check which bits of brain to leave alone and which to remove. Counting was strange. I was asked to count forwards and backwards and found that I couldn't do it, then I could, then I couldn't again. From time to time I could hear a bit of the drilling and scraping. That was a weird sensation."
> Richard Stevens

What if I can't have surgery?

Some patients, including myself, have been told that their tumours are inoperable. In my case, my brain tumour is located in the left frontal lobe and diffuses into parts of my brain responsible for language processing and movement on my right hand side. My early brain surgeons and neurologists agreed that it would be too dangerous to attempt surgery in these areas. Later brain surgeons have disagreed, saying they might be able to operate safely. For the time being, my wife and I have decided not to risk brain surgery. It will always be your own decision as to whether to proceed or not.

If you cannot have brain surgery, your oncologist will want you to have a biopsy. They will take a number of samples of your tumour, from the parts they are most concerned about and that they can get to safely. They will then test these samples, to look at the shape of their cells and their genetic makeup. They will then be able to give you a histology, telling you the type and grade of tumour you have. The results will guide your oncologist's next steps.

A biopsy is a form of brain surgery, and it takes place under anaesthetic. As with full brain surgery, you may have stickers put onto your face and head, and a metal frame attached to your skull if the surgeon needs the help of computer guidance to reach the tumour. A small piece of skull will be drilled away, perhaps a hole 1cm across, and then a computer guided needle will be used to remove small parts your tumour. Once done, your skull will either be replaced or a piece of metal, a wire mesh or a plastic plug may be placed in the hole before your skin is sewn up. You may still end up with a sizeable scar, and a deep dimple in your skull where the incision was made.

What can surgery achieve?

For brain tumours, surgery can be effective in the short term. Soon after surgery, perhaps even within days or weeks, you'll be given an MRI scan to see what impact the surgery has had on the tumour and its surrounding brain tissue, and to check for any swelling and pooling of liquid. In extreme circumstances, your surgeon may wish to try surgery again – particularly if swelling, movement or growth in the tumour means they may be able to get more of it out. Otherwise, you're likely to be given some time to rest before the next stages of your treatment are planned.

Brain surgery is not the only or whole solution to anaplastic astrocytoma and glioblastoma. That is why it will always be backed up with a combination of radiotherapy and chemotherapy, to attempt to attack any remaining cancer cells in the brain. As you are coming to learn, astrocytoma cancers are very hardy. Even a few cells left in the brain after surgery can lead to brain tumour reoccurrence. Since brain tumours are made up of millions of cells, total resection – the complete removal of a tumour – is unlikely. In a diffuse tumour, your surgeon has an enormous job to follow each of the tentacles, taking out the cancerous cells from each part of the brain into which they have leaked. Some surgical research and progress is being done at a number of cancer centres worldwide with a substance called 5-ALA, which a patient drinks before they go into surgery. This makes cancerous cells glow pink under ultraviolet light, and helps the surgeon to chase after migrating glioblastoma cells.

With a diffuse tumour it is very likely that the tumour will have gone into parts of the brain that cannot be cut away to get at the cancerous cells. To do so would affect the patient's language, movement, cognitive skills or natural body responses like breathing, sight and hearing. Surgeons won't cut away a tumour where it puts other brain functions at risk. (We might like to make that decision for them, but their Hippocratic oath to 'do no harm' prevents them from seriously damaging one part of our ability, to save another).

That does not mean surgery should not take place. Reducing the size of the tumour can have a significant effect on progression free survival, and on overall survival for patients. It can free up pressure in the brain and, complemented by radiotherapy and chemotherapy, can put a very real stop to brain tumour growth for months and even years.

And a single surgery isn't always the only option. Some patients have two, three or even more surgeries in response to the growth of their tumour. The ultimate aim will always be to extend life, while not putting basic functionality at risk. As medical science improves, more is becoming possible for brain tumour patients, meaning things believed impossible in brain surgery even 10 years ago are regularly taking place. The hope is that surgeons can keep brain tumour patients alive long enough to reap the benefits of continually evolving techniques and new research.

> "George's surgeon likened the cancer cells to a battlefield. After the massacre of the tumour – he'd achieved over 95% resection – he was unsure how many of the bloodied, wounded cells would lay down and die, and how many would grow stronger and regroup and needed further attack. We were advised to undergo radiation and temozolomide chemotherapy. George was entered into a trial and was randomly selected to have radiation alongside chemotherapy, and then chemotherapy for a year. We felt it the right thing to hit it hard."
> Jane Cooke, mother of George

Whether to go for surgery or not, and at what particular time, is probably more of an art than a science. Even among brain surgeons. My story mirrors Duncan Weaver's again in that we were both put on a watch and wait protocol, and we were both satisfied to see how things developed. And like mine, Duncan's doctors could never seem to get his seizures under control. Even after two years of changing and increasing medication.

Eventually Duncan's neurologist in the Netherlands sent his case for review. The board of review were in two minds, and sent Duncan for a further opinion in Rotterdam. Neither Duncan nor Loes expected surgery to be recommended. After all, Duncan's was still a low grade brain tumour. They had both decided to get on with their lives. They were delighted that Loes was seven months pregnant.

But in the waiting room, Duncan began to waver. He turned to his expectant wife and whispered what had obviously been on his mind: "Just be prepared that he might say we actually need to do the operation now."

When the appointment came, the neurosurgeon did exactly that. New practice was to take out even low grade brain tumours as soon as possible, and since Duncan's had shown some activity (on a single scan, which didn't appear on subsequent ones), now was the best time to act.

By 'now', the surgeon meant within a month or two. Just about the time Loes was due to give birth. For Duncan that wasn't going to work. He'd rather put his health at risk than not be there when his baby was born. In the end, Duncan negotiated with the doctor to have an awake craniotomy just six weeks after his baby girl Tess came into the world.

James Campling had an awake craniotomy at the John Radcliffe Hospital in Oxford, England in July, less than a month since the fateful journey across Finland.

It was a seven hour slog, for much of which he was kept awake. But things didn't go as well as was hoped. The brain tumour had infiltrated into both verbal and motor areas of his brain, so it could not be fully removed. Also during surgery James had a massive seizure; his entire body shaking and putting the whole operation at risk.

It might be time to close him up, the surgeon suggested, but James wanted the operation to continue. Despite the seizure, his military training had taught him the logic of continuing now so as to prevent having to have more operations later on. The surgeon continued.

Over the next few days, James and his family met with the surgeon and oncologist at the hospital to discuss the results. James had a glioblastoma.

The surgeon had managed to remove the majority of it, but he now had an infection that needed attention. The operation had also cut into James's language area, so his ability to speak properly was curtailed in the short term. He would have to relearn how to speak, and take a longer recovery period than he had hoped for.

Once he had recovered, James would have to start chemotherapy and radiotherapy. More surgery might be needed in the future. If it was what the science recommended, then James wanted it. He knew it couldn't last, but that thought was liberating in a way.

He'd never have to worry about a pension or old age. He could live out the years to come pursuing the adventures he'd dreamed of.

So James was determined to make the most of his recovery, and he took every opportunity to get fitter again following his recovery period. Just as his chemotherapy began, James was able to run a hilly marathon with friends over the Yorkshire peaks in aid of Brain Tumour Research. He also took time to travel with his mum to Belarus.

The side effects of surgery

Brain surgery itself is considered quite safe, or at least no more risky than other major surgery on vital organs. But you may be disappointed when you first come round that everything is not functioning as you'd hoped. Your language may be confused, you'll probably feel nauseous, your movement may be restricted and your seizures may be more frequent than before.

It is likely this will be due to inflammation and bruising from the operation, rather than some critical injury to part of the brain. Within a relatively short time, your condition should settle of its own accord or with steroids that may be given to you following surgery.

However, that's not always the case. Some patients do not recover from surgery well, or find they have developed some longer term cognition and ability restrictions as a result; they may be passed to a language therapist or physiotherapist to help them relearn or develop some of the skills that may have become restricted.

Common short term side effects from surgery include any of the following: weakness, nausea, poor balance, dizziness, change in personality, fatigue, and sight and hearing loss. This is all a normal part of the surgery process, and you and your family should not worry unduly unless your doctors express concern.

> "I had already seen a lot of atrophy [loss of strength] through my left side before surgery and was expected to encounter some substantial motor control deficits. Thankfully none manifested in quite that fashion because I had a great surgeon who carried out an awake craniotomy. A number of things turned off internally, I received some facial paralysis and my palate disengaged, alongside some bladder control issues (which I was thankfully well versed in thanks to the seizures, but it isn't great for your social life). The large part of my physicality has remained intact though, which has been great."
> Jack Webb

More worrying side effects of brain surgery may be stroke, serious swelling along the ventricles of the brain, or a build up or leak of fluid from the cerebral spinal fluid. Your surgeon will need to act accordingly to deal with these outcomes.

Many brain tumour patients find they have to have some kind of rehabilitation after surgery, and it is likely you will see an occupational therapist who is responsible for looking at your home and working life, and helping you and others adapt to your limitations, whether temporary or permanent.

"Sue went for a biopsy in May, and we were elated when the consultant told her that it was an astrocytoma, and not a glioblastoma. He was extremely optimistic about treatment. But she'd gained a bleed on the brain as a result of the biopsy, and had to stay in hospital for two weeks instead of a few days. Had we known these risks beforehand we would never have had the biopsy done."

Joanna Waters, sister of Sue Rossides

Even though Duncan Weaver's first surgery was to remove a low grade tumour, it was not without difficulty. While his wife, his six week old daughter and family waited at home and the hospital, Duncan underwent a five hour open craniotomy.

Like James Campling, he was awoken during the operation for around 90 minutes to be asked questions and urged to move parts of his body so the surgeon could avoid motor and speech areas.

And like James, Duncan's movement on one side appeared to have been severely affected. At first, he assumed it would be short term. But doctors were concerned that the paralysis was lasting and he would need rehabilitation to use his right leg, foot, arm and hand again. In total, Duncan spent seven weeks in rehabilitation for his physical mobility.

His right foot became what is impolitely called 'drop foot', essentially a numb limb which Duncan had to drag around with him while walking. He carried a stick for balance and support, as the strength in his right leg had diminished. He regained the use of his arm, though full feeling didn't return even after physiotherapy. Neither Duncan's right leg, arm or hand worked properly unless he was looking at them, a weird sensation but a known condition called proprioception. It also caused his limbs to wander, which could be dangerous when Duncan was trying to cook.

It was a tough time for the couple. Though they had been told about the risks of surgery, they of course didn't want him to be in that small percentage of patients that emerge from theatre with lasting disability. It was particularly tough because of the timing of Tess's birth. The rehab centre had brought him a long way since surgery, but it would never be able to do everything.

True to type, the couple decided to take the setback in their stride. They would have to concentrate not on what Duncan couldn't do anymore, but instead on what he could. Play to his strengths.

And anyway, analysis of his tumour had shown Duncan still had a low grade astrocytoma. There was a long way to go yet. His doctors still suggested there could be up to 20 years of life after treatment.

But before the road to recovery could really begin, Duncan had to go into the next stage of his treatment: radiotherapy.

Radiotherapy

"As soon as we found out that it was a Grade III oligoastrocytoma tumour I was contending with, my doctors advised me to start a treatment plan of 30 sessions of radiotherapy, followed by a four week rest and then straight into 12 rounds of temozolomide chemotherapy. I doubled down on the research and made a detailed list of questions to take to my meetings. At the end of the day, I ended up going down the path that the oncologists were suggesting, but I wanted to be sure that it was the right treatment for me. I wanted to feel as though I was in control of the situation, that it was on my terms."

Calum Wright

It is very likely that your oncologist will advise radiotherapy for the treatment of your brain tumour. You'll either be encouraged to have it immediately after surgery, or after a period of watch and wait.

With anaplastic astrocytomas and glioblastomas, the World Health Organization suggests concurrent radiotherapy and chemotherapy as soon after surgery as possible. More and more doctors are recommending early radiotherapy for other brain tumours too, as research is suggesting better outcomes this way.

You may find the idea of radiotherapy unpleasant or something to be afraid of, but it can be effective for many subtypes of anaplastic astrocytoma and glioblastoma.

The radiotherapy regime your oncologist will recommend you follow is most likely to be for the maximum level of radiation, for six weeks. It is most likely to be the type of radiotherapy called fractionated external beam radiation therapy (EBRT). The 'fractionated' aspect is that treatment is split into a number of different doses, delivered over a number of weeks. The treatment is high powered X-rays, directed at the tumour from outside the body.

This type of radiotherapy, like other types, delivers high doses of X-rays very directly to the tumour cells, where they disrupt the DNA of the cancer cells. They die off and are unable to reproduce, destroying the tumour. Meanwhile, the surrounding healthy brain tissue is kept as intact as possible. Radiotherapy can be very accurate: the shape of the tumour can be 'cut out' by the radiation beams, even if it is quite sprawling. The beams are fired into your brain at different depths, creating a 3D attack on the tumour.

To ensure as much of the tumour as possible is targeted, your oncologist and therapeutic radiologist will very specifically plan your treatment. They will use your MRI scans to map your tumour, or what is left of it after surgery. They will add an extra margin of up to 3cm around the tumour, to try to capture any brain tumour cells that have infiltrated into surrounding tissue.

Patients are often astounded to see their first or second MRI after radiation, because their tumour often seems to have disappeared completely. This shows the effectiveness of radiation at destroying tumours in many cases, though you should be clear that it is not always successful. Some glioblastomas in particular seem to be hardly affected by radiation, or else grow back very quickly afterwards.

One accusation often levelled at radiation is that it can actually speed up the regrowth of brain tumours. So far, there is no evidence that this is the case. Much more likely is that the patients for whom tumours quickly return after radiation already had very fast growing tumours, or that oncologists recommended radiotherapy because they detected rapid growth but did not communicate this well enough to their patients. This is a real concern among patients, and oncologists should make more effort to reassure them. We patients also need to ask the right questions.

Unless you are particularly claustrophobic or suffer from panic attacks, radiotherapy is not especially unpleasant. In fact, you will find it very much like a shorter version of an MRI scan, but with much more space. Occasionally, your radiological team will build some scans into your radiotherapy (to ensure correct positioning). The difference is a radiotherapy machine is nowhere near as noisy as an MRI.

But you will need to wear a tight fitting mask during treatment. If you find wearing an MRI headset unpleasant, you may initially struggle with a radiotherapy mask because they're very close and tight fitting indeed.

Having your mask fitted is the first step in fractionated EBRT. This I found the most unpleasant aspect of all of my radiotherapy. The fitting takes place in two stages.

You will be invited to lie on a couch with your head and shoulders exposed. Technicians will then place a sheet of plastic mesh into a vat of hot water. The plastic becomes flexible, and will be laid over your face, head and neck. Quickly, they will expand the small hole already in the middle of the mesh to create a space for your mouth and nose. You'll be able to breathe normally.

Next, they will press the mesh around your face, so as to create a tight fit around your face and head. Already, you'll begin to feel the mask harden. The technologists will then use plastic clips to fasten the newly made mask to the headboard you're lying on, creating a very snug fit. Finally, they may switch on some fans blowing cold air until the plastic turns into a solid, tight fitting mask that resembles your face.

That's your mask made, and time for a rest. They'll quickly unclip you from the bench and release you back into the waiting room, or most likely say you can go home. Depending on how quickly your oncologist wants things moving, a technical team will now use your MRI scans to map your mask, creating areas where the radiation beams should be allowed to enter your skull, and marking other areas with reflective tape to prevent beams from getting through.

An alternative to this process is the creation of a kind of papier-mâché version of your head, where the technicians will lay strips of bandages, wetted with plaster across your face. Once dry, they will use this as a mould for creating a perspex mask.

When you next see your mask, it will be covered in markings, which will correspond to coordinates in the radiotherapy computer. You will then have to be properly aligned with the radiotherapy machine, and it's this part I found most uncomfortable. At your first radiotherapy appointment, you will be asked to lie on the bench again and the mask will be fastened tightly to the bench, holding your head very still. Unlike in an MRI machine, where you might be making a conscious effort not to move your head, in a radiotherapy machine you won't be *able* to move.

There will then begin a good half hour of calibrating: you, the markings on your mask, and the radiotherapy machine together. The machine operators will continually come into the room to make adjustments to the tape on the mask, and to draw on it with a marker pen.

But it is not like an MRI machine. You are not fed into a doughnut. Instead a machine with two giant limbs rotates around you from a distance of about a metre. From the patient's perspective, you'll see light beams move around, as the operators make very slight adjustments to the bench's height and angles. What the technicians are doing is ensuring that every time you are clipped onto the bench – up to 30 times over the next six weeks – your head will be in exactly the same position, and that the radiotherapy beams entering your brain will be in exactly the same place, reaching exactly the same depth.

But fitting is not an easy job. By 15 minutes of this, I was fed up and felt restricted and frustrated. After half an hour, I wasn't sure if I could take any more and almost pressed the panic button to ask for a rest. But by telling myself that the process had to stop soon, I managed to get through it. And stop it eventually did.

I was grateful to be told by the technician that the actual therapy was nowhere near as difficult as the mask fitting, and this turned out to be true. Every subsequent treatment had my head snapped back onto that bench for no more than eight or nine minutes each time. The machine rotated, and the bed on which I lay rotated, but the discomfort was always very short lived.

Radiotherapy treatment doesn't hurt. You will not feel anything during the short treatment itself at all. I cycled five miles to and from every one of my radiotherapy treatments, without feeling any negative effects. During radiotherapy, your technician will leave you alone in the room with the machine, but will monitor you through an observation window and most likely by intercom too. You'll be up and back in the waiting room before you've even had time to get bored.

Every couple of weeks, you may be given a contrast dye drip (just as in an MRI scan), so that pictures can be taken while you are under the machine. These images of your tumour are to ensure that the radiotherapy is still being directed at exactly the right place, rather than to monitor the progress of the treatment. You may also be given steroids, to keep swelling at bay while your tumour is zapped, as well as anti-sickness drugs.

There are other types of radiotherapy which your doctors might consider. You may also have heard of gamma knife, stereotactic, and proton beam radiotherapy. These are developing fields and are not yet considered realistic prospects for very diffuse and fast growing brain tumours like anaplastic astrocytoma and glioblastoma in adults.

Lian's mother went into surgery with a doctor she had researched thoroughly, and had been recommended to the family. For Lian, researching on the internet had positive and negative results.

Negative, because no matter where she looked, the ultimate result of the brain tumour her mother had was always the same. This was really happening, and there was little anyone could do about it.

But positive too, not only because she discovered a burgeoning community of brain tumour patients and loved ones online from whom she could gather information, but also because she found out that new clinical trials were coming on stream all the time. New treatments were being developed. It gave her hope not for a cure, but for more time and a better outcome for her mum.

The surgery went well, but Lian wasn't surprised to learn the surgeon hadn't been able to remove all of the tumour. But he'd been able to take out a very large chunk, which meant the radiotherapy and chemotherapy Gillian had to begin immediately had a better chance of being effective.

When Lian's mother had her radiotherapy mask fitted, to Lian it looked like something out of a horror film. She could barely watch. Just seeing the finished mask made her feel sick. She clung to the idea that this ordeal was going to work in the end, keeping the tumour away for as long as possible.

Duncan Weaver's experience of radiotherapy was pretty typical. He had 28 sessions, five days a week. The daily grind of attending each session was very tiring, and he could be travelling and then waiting for three hours just for a 10 minute appointment. But the first three weeks went without mishap.

He then began to lose his hair, so reverted to the short crop he'd had at university and he and Loes soon got used to it. But from the end of week three, radiotherapy began to get hard every day. Duncan started getting very tired, having to sleep each afternoon as soon as he returned from treatment. That meant he couldn't spend time with his new daughter, nor make the most of Christmas and New Year which fell during treatment.

It was a time for Duncan and Loes to pull together. Loes made an advent calendar, counting down the days to the last session. That final Friday afternoon they looked towards a bigger celebration than Christmas and New Year put together.

Chemotherapy

It is very likely that you will be advised to take

chemotherapy either alongside or immediately after surgery and radiotherapy on your brain tumour. There are a number of accepted and effective chemotherapy regimes for brain tumours of different types. The breed and even genetic signature of your brain tumour will dictate the one that is most likely to work for you.

As always, your oncologist will be seeking to offer the most effective treatment for your tumour, taking into account how well you tolerate the drugs. These drugs are toxic – that's why they work. Their toxicity can also have profound negative effects on your body, and some find them intolerable. In some cases, patients just feel so sick, incapacitated or poorly affected by the chemotherapy that they cannot proceed. In the first instance, doctors are likely to try you on a different type of chemo that might be slightly less effective but better tolerated.

Temozolomide

> "I had six cycles of chemo, temozolomide. I did feel more tired than normal while taking the pills but otherwise not too bad. Just as you are starting to feel better at the end of the cycle, bang – you start on the next one."
> Richard Stevens

If you have an anaplastic astrocytoma or a glioblastoma, the most frequently used chemotherapy drug used is called temozolomide. In the UK the marketing name for it is Temodal; in the US it is called Temodar.

Most brain tumours of these types receive temozolomide, but not all. That's because for those few patients with particular genetic signatures in their tumours, the drug isn't considered effective enough to justify the toxicity. One of the key ways temozolomide is effective is in intensifying the power of radiotherapy. You are likely to take it while you are having radiotherapy, because the two work better together than by themselves. This is called chemoradiation or chemoradiotherapy.

Temozolomide is a type of chemotherapy that circulates in the blood stream, though it is taken as a tablet. It is a cytotoxic drug, meaning it is a drug that kills cells. Because this particular drug can cross the blood-brain barrier – a gateway that can prevent other diseases and viruses from getting to the brain – it is often used to treat brain tumours.

Your oncologist will design and plan the most appropriate temozolomide treatment for you, depending on your tumour, your weight, your reaction to the drug, fatigue levels and other factors.

The drug is a capsule that you take once a day, usually over an hour before meals. If you're having radiotherapy at the same time, you may be asked to take it before each treatment, throughout treatment.

A typical course of temozolomide *after* radiotherapy may see you then take the drug for five days every four weeks, for six cycles of treatment. During this time, you'll probably see your oncologist once per cycle to report any side effects. You may also be given an emergency telephone number, in case of some sudden negative reaction to the drug. There are a number of negative side effects to temozolomide. Their severity varies from patient to patient, and in some patients the reaction is so pronounced they are unable to continue the treatment.

"After my surgery was drug time. There were the usual six weeks of radiotherapy and chemo. I was assigned temozolomide. The first round was just six weeks, and it was okay. Some days I slept a lot more than usual, but the weeks passed reasonably quickly. Then I had to have another series, lasting for six months with the drug increasing each month. But it affected me badly. In month four I was advised by my oncologist the tumour had not shrunk. Temozolomide was not working."
Graham Dunnett

Other types of chemotherapy

If you are unable to continue temozolomide, your oncologist will consider a different chemotherapy that may be more tolerable for you. Often this will depend on the country, or even the region or hospital, where you are being treated. Currently in the UK, for example, those who tolerate temozolomide poorly may be considered for PCV treatment, a type of chemotherapy that uses a combination of drugs.

Under PCV, you will receive three different drugs, potentially for six cycles, each cycle lasting six weeks. On day one you receive vincristine, a chemotherapy drug that is delivered through a drip in hospital. You will also be given lomustine, another powerful chemotherapy drug. You will then be sent home to take a third chemotherapy drug that evening, procarbazine. You'll also get steroids and anti-sickness drugs. For the next nine days you'll take procarbazine in the evening. The remaining four weeks are 'rest and recovery', though my experience of PCV chemotherapy is that it hits hardest in weeks three and four. It's a complex cocktail, and the first drug, vincristine, is so toxic it has to be kept in an opaque bag so it doesn't react with light.

In the US, oncologists will often revert to a combination of two drugs, carmustine and lomustine. If you have surgery, they may place into your brain a 'Gliadel wafer', a sliver of drug that will gradually dissolve around the tumour. The insertion of these wafers is becoming less common, as more effective chemotherapy and radiotherapy treatments make the effort and risk required less worth taking.

In the United States you may also be offered bevacizumab (Avastin) as part of a trial. This aims to starve tumours of blood by disrupting angiogenesis, the generation of tumour blood vessels. The most recent summary of research concluded that it is not considered effective in treating glioblastomas, but there are ongoing trials and research projects.[11] It is not available in the UK, but if you have a generous health insurer they may pay for you to go to the United States for treatment.

These are by no means all the chemotherapy options available for anaplastic astrocytoma and glioblastoma, they are simply those most often used. Others are available and are being tested, and you may be asked or able to join one of the trials of a drug even if it isn't yet approved as an official treatment for brain tumours. Your doctors and oncologists will advise.

The immediate side effects of treatment

Some side effects you'll begin to feel right away. Others will emerge over the weeks, as the treatment really kicks in. The thing to remember here is that, in many cases, experiencing side effects means the treatment is doing what it should be.

Fatigue

The real problem with cancer treatment is the repetition. You are likely to have up to 30 radiotherapy treatments, for example: once a day, five days a week, for six weeks. Only the weekends will offer you a break. Simply hauling yourself to the hospital every day, particularly if you are coming from far away, can be draining.

While some are able to continue working or home life normally during treatment, the reality is that most have to give their lives over to treatment while it lasts and put everything else on hold. Even if your treatment lasts for just 10 minutes, you might find yourself waiting for a couple of hours or more each day for it to begin.

If you are having chemotherapy at the same time, the continual treatment, waiting and travel can create enormous tiredness and physical fatigue. The drugs you'll be given for chemotherapy will also create fatigue, with or without radiotherapy.

Some hospitals offer the opportunity to stay on site or close by during treatment, either for free or at low cost. Medical insurers may pay for a local hotel, understanding that the real impact of treatment is not the whizz-burr of treatment itself, but the daily grind of travel and stress for six weeks.

Hair loss

You can expect to lose some hair during radiotherapy where the X-rays enter and exit your skull, and this may not grow back fully or even the same colour or texture after treatment is complete. But radiotherapy isn't likely to lead to the all over alopecia like hair loss that is the popular picture of a cancer patient.

Some chemotherapy regimes are also known to lead to hair loss, though neither temozolomide nor PCV are regarded as being among them, though they might thin out your hair.

One year on from my radiotherapy, I still have a large patch of missing hair where the beams went into my head, and a smaller one where the beams left the other side of my skull. It means I tend to keep the rest of my hair very short all over. Balding anyway, my hair loss is not a significant factor for me, but I don't underestimate the impact it has on many women, as well as some men who before treatment could boast far more impressive locks than I ever could.

Infection

During your chemotherapy, you'll be asked to try to avoid colds, infections and viruses because your ability to fight everyday infections will be hugely reduced. Of course, that's easier said than done, particularly if you're trying to stay at work, if you have young children sharing bugs around at school, or if you have lots of visitors.

Chemotherapy attacks both your white and red blood cells. The former are responsible for fighting infections, so a low white blood cell count means even the start of a common cold could make you more susceptible to pneumonia if it is not brought into line quickly. A reduced red blood cell count means your blood might not clot as well as it should, meaning cuts, bruises and burns might not heal and might become infected more easily. Damage to either type of blood cell count is bound to contribute to fatigue.

Your doctors will ask you to have frequent tests to 'check your bloods'. They will want to ensure your white and red blood cell counts are high enough to allow you to proceed with the next round of chemotherapy, for example. This is because giving you chemo while your blood defences are already weak will weaken your immune system yet further, leading to severe vulnerability to dangerous infection.

Dry, frazzled skin

When you introduce radiation to your skin, it is just like going out in the sun too long. Your skin is likely to get a little fried as the beams pass through. Unfortunately, you can't just slap on the sunscreen as you would by the seaside, because that would prevent the radiation from getting through. Instead, your radiotherapy team will give you a decent moisturiser to apply to anywhere that's beginning to feel sore. After radiotherapy, sunscreen is a must if you're going out in direct sunlight.

Seizures

You may find radiotherapy has a profound effect on your seizure patterns, initially increasing (or even beginning) the number of seizures you have. This is because the treatment can lead to scarring and to inflammation in the brain, causing abnormal activity in those brain areas. In the medium term, though, radiotherapy aims to shrink your brain tumour, and any negative effects that go with it, including seizures.

In my own experience, my seizures seemed to stop

almost overnight as soon as I began radiotherapy. Before I began, I was having them 10, 20, even 30 times a day. Once the radiation began, those light seizures disappeared to almost nothing. Nearly six months from the end of my radiation, I can report that they don't seem to have returned in any huge way. It's possible, of course, that a change in drugs contributed to the reduction in seizures too.

Nausea

After around three weeks of radiotherapy I began to feel mildly nauseous. By week five, I was nauseous most of the time. So much so that I lost my appetite, and spent my time nibbling on dry crackers instead of eating bigger meals.

But it was after the radiotherapy finished that I really would feel sick, often into the evenings. Though I never actually threw up, it was clear the nausea was down to the radiotherapy because I wasn't having chemotherapy at the same time. If you are having temozolomide as well as radiotherapy, the likelihood of nausea is very high.

Many patients are sick and are given anti-sickness medication (called 'antiemetics') as well as steroids, to keep the sickness at bay.

Constipation

It is a cruel twist of cancer treatment that the drugs you'll receive to reduce your nausea may at the same time give you severe constipation. Your team will give you laxatives and through personal experience I'd advise you to get onto them as soon as you start taking anti-sickness drugs.

Don't kid yourself that eating figs or dried apple

will do the job just as well. Oral laxative tastes awful, no matter how 'orange flavoured' the box might claim it to be. But the alternative is long and painful stints on the toilet that become really quite unpleasant. Your chemotherapy may cause constipation also, so you might as well throw in your lot, take a deep breath, and get the laxative down you.

The long term effects of radiotherapy

Before beginning radiation, your oncologist should go over the long term effects of the treatment with you. It is a fact that radiotherapy can create new brain tumours in the medium to long term. But evidence suggests this is very infrequent and almost always many years – decades – after radiation has taken place.

The brain tumours created do not have any relation to the original brain tumour that radiation intended to treat. As such, the new tumours, if they occur at all, may be benign, removable or independently treatable.

Because radiotherapy can also cause brain cell death in the longer term, it can lead to delayed side effects over many years such as memory loss, slower brain function, higher risk of stroke or stroke like symptoms, and personality changes. All of these long term effects are considered of low probability and are secondary to the immediate need to treat your brain tumour.

At any time during your brain tumour journey, whether before you are even diagnosed or when you are reacting or recovering from surgery or treatment, you may feel unwell.

Apart from the key signs and symptoms of brain

tumours already covered, and the main side effects of treatment, there are a few other health problems you may wish to look out for. Simply having a tumour is no excuse for feeling unwell, and your doctor will try to make you as comfortable as you can be. But they do need to know the symptoms you are experiencing.

Swelling

You may feel the build up of liquid in the brain, the skull, or elsewhere in the central nervous system such as the spine, as an increased feeling of pressure or severe head or muscle ache. If you are uncomfortable, your doctor may seek to relieve some of this swelling by inserting a tube, called a shunt, to drain off some fluid. They may prescribe some steroids which can reduce swelling.

Blood clots

These can be quite common in people with high grade gliomas. Up to a third of patients may develop a deep vein blood clot, according to the National Comprehensive Cancer Network (NCNN) in the United States.[12] The clot is potentially harmful, because it could block a vein in our lungs. Symptoms include swelling, skin redness and discomfort in the limbs.

Endocrine disorders

The NCNN also warns of health problems relating to your hormone system, which a brain tumour can influence. Look out for a general feeling of being unwell and your doctor will be able to asses if your hormones are working as they should.

Novel treatments

Surgery, chemotherapy and radiotherapy – usually combined – are by far the most effective and frequently used forms of treatment for these types of brain tumours. But that's not the end of the story. Many brain tumour and cancer centres across the world are developing, testing and rolling out other forms of treatment that have built upon traditional treatments.

Some surgeons and oncologists consider some of these 'cutting edge' techniques as fads or fashion, while others swear by their efficacy. What's important to remember as patients is that in most cases, the technology is so new and brain tumours are so complex, that the jury is still out.

Novel treatments are often a good option to pursue when other treatments have not worked or have stopped working. However, due consideration should always be given to their scientific and medical viability, as well as their probability of being useful to patients. Unfortunately, the world of cancer features far too many 'quacks' out to make money or achieve fame, and unproven 'cures' which are nothing of the kind.

You should only undertake a novel treatment or clinical trial if it has been approved by your own country or region's national medical and ethical advisory boards.

And you should consider very carefully before travelling to countries that are not known to have robust medical oversight of trials, in order to get some mystery or miracle treatment. If it looks too good to be true, it probably is.

It is advised you always consult your own doctors and oncologists before beginning any kind of treatment. Of course you're bound to consult the internet, but always sense test any proposed treatment or cure with medical professionals and ask them for their honest opinion. To get a full picture, the more professional cancer experts you can consult the better.

Saying that, developments in brain tumour treatment are happening all the time. This book will quickly fall out of date as research continues apace. That's a good thing.

The following are considered cutting edge, developing treatments that are being routinely used to treat and tackle serious brain tumours. Usually, they'd be used when routine surgery, chemotherapy and radiotherapy have been tried first. No-one is yet guaranteeing success from any of these treatments, but there have been some promising results in terms of extending or improving quality of life.

Gamma knife / stereotactic radiotherapy

These are specific types of radiotherapy, also known as 'radiosurgery', but are only suitable for very small brain tumours. Under this treatment, very targeted beams of radiation 'cut out' the 3D shape of the tumour from your brain. They are not suitable for tumours that have diffused into the surrounding brain tissue. Unfortunately, the technology is not routinely used for anaplastic astrocytoma or glioblastoma because these tumours are often large and diffuse. Recurring tumours might be treated with gamma knife when they first return and are still small (called 'salvage stereotactic radiosurgery').

Proton beam therapy (PBT)

This works the same way as traditional

radiotherapy, except that very fast moving protons are fired at the tumour cells. Unlike the X-rays used in radiotherapy, the energised particle proton beams are stopped by the tumour so cannot penetrate very far. This means the tumour gets the biggest hit from the treatment, while the rest of the brain – particularly further into the brain, behind the tumour – receives less radiation than in conventional radiotherapy.

It is currently considered suitable for very few patients, though the field is fast developing. It is unlikely to be offered to patients with large and diffuse tumours, as it wouldn't work effectively. That's because it needs to 'cut' an accurate line around the tumour, and diffuse tumours just don't have this break where brain ends and tumour begins. Adults are only likely to be able to access proton beam therapy as part of a medical trial. It is not available in the UK, though plans are afoot.

The therapy needs to be delivered alongside (rather than instead of) chemotherapy, takes a long time because of its very precise nature, and for patients in the UK can only be accessed abroad. The Brain Tumour Charity in the UK says that the process for being referred abroad by the NHS takes a long time and so delays possible treatment, which may not be in the patients' interests.

They also say that going to private centres abroad means the child or adult may not be given chemotherapy alongside the PBT, and so delays this aspect of their treatment. This may result in less intensive treatment and reduced tumour control.

Immunotherapy
This is one of a number of types of 'biologic' or

'targeted' therapies. Biologic therapies aim to disrupt the normal behaviour of brain tumour cells, say by preventing the biological pathways these cells rely on to reproduce or fight your body's natural defences.

Immunotherapy is a specific type of this targeted therapy, and is one of the latest good news prospects in cancer treatment – particularly in brain tumours. It concentrates on how your body normally attacks foreign or irregular cells, and how brain tumour cells try to prevent these attacks. By using drugs, it deactivates the defence mechanisms of brain tumour cells, and upscales your natural immune system's attacks on infection.

In this way immunotherapy supports your own body to attack the tumour. Immunotherapy is considered one of the most cutting edge potential treatments for glioblastoma. There are a number of trials, and in some cases it is the natural next step if temozolomide is not suitable or has not worked.

Virus therapies

Some researchers are examining how to use elements of viruses such as polio or herpes to spread in the body and naturally attack brain tumour cells, though this treatment is in its infancy.

Gene editing

The whole area of genes and brain tumours is very new, with so much still unknown about the genetic makeup of brain tumours, and the gene processes involved in their growth, resistance and death. One promising avenue of research is attacking brain tumours at the genetic level, or changing genes in the body's immune system to destroy brain tumour cells.

So what is my doctor looking for?

After surgery and treatment, your oncologist and surgeon will mainly be looking at images of your brain to monitor progress.

Initially, particularly after radiotherapy, they may not be able to see much. This is because surgery and radiotherapy cause scarring and swelling in the brain. It is hard to see what has changed, because *so much* will have. Comparing MRI scans to the pre-treatment brain might be a red herring, because apart from showing that the tumour may have shrunk or gone into hiding, it is otherwise difficult to get a good picture. Most oncologists will seek to take a 'baseline' scan after radiotherapy, and then each MRI afterwards will be compared against this baseline to see how the post-treatment brain is behaving.

So, what will they be looking for? First, any dangerous swelling as a result of the radiotherapy. The treatment can cause pockets of oedema (build up of fluid) that can put pressure on the brain and cause its own tumour like symptoms. They may decide surgery or a thin draining tube (called a 'shunt') might need to be inserted to relieve the pressure. You may have a shunt remaining from surgery.

Second, they'll be seeking the tumour itself. Has it shrunk? Is there evidence of any malignant cells remaining? Your doctors will want to see how any remaining cancer cells are behaving. This is why you will have radiotherapy, then chemotherapy, or both at the same time: to catch those remaining cells. It's very possible that remaining cells will be dying off, but very unlikely that every cancer cell will disappear completely. Treatment could well 'knock back' your tumour, but it will not cure it. Your physician will want to monitor whatever remains closely to detect any new growth early.

Which means the third aspect your doctors will be looking for is so-called recurrence of the tumour. This is new growth either where the tumour previously was, or from any cancer cells surviving following your treatment. Obviously, if rapid regrowth occurs between MRIs they'll want to act accordingly. That might mean more surgery, more chemotherapy or in very rare cases more radiotherapy.

In this intervening time, you will be asked to keep a very close eye on your brain tumour symptoms. An increase in seizures, nausea, headaches, language problems or confusion could be indicative of tumour regrowth, though it's important to state that they don't definitely herald it. This is made all the more confusing if you are having ongoing treatment, because radiotherapy and chemotherapy makes these symptoms worse before they, hopefully, go away.

'Watch and wait' after treatment

> "Of course he complained of being bored, wanted a job, wanted more, but he had to balance the long term fatigue and chemo with all he wanted to do. But overall when I said to him 'George, is there anything special you want to do?' he said, 'Mum, I just want to live my usual everyday life.'"
> Jane Cooke, mother of George

Unfortunately for some anaplastic astrocytoma and glioblastoma patients, it will feel like they are in some kind of cancer treatment – or recovering from it – for the rest of their lives.

Yet for many patients, there will be long periods ranging from a month to three months, six months or even longer after treatment when they will be sent home while doctors 'watch and wait' for the results to show themselves, or for something else to happen.

On the surface, this is of course to be welcomed. Not being in treatment will be more welcome than being in hospital or recovering in pain, nausea or being constipated. But at the same time, it can generate a feeling of being lost, not knowing what is going on inside your head, fearing for the future and judging every little headache or missed word as an indication that something serious is about to occur.

It doesn't help that these periods have become known in the brain tumour community as 'watch and wait', as both words imply fear. Watch: never take your eye off the ball, never forget you have a brain tumour. Wait: this thing will get you in the end, and your job is simply to wait helplessly for it to do so.

Patients can often feel depressed at this time. First, they are bound to fear the future and what it might bring. This anxiety can be stifling, and take over your ability to live day to day. As your next MRI scan and results day approaches, this anxiety can be ramped up as you begin to imagine what you are about to be told and its implications.

But there can also be a feeling of uselessness in this period. For brain tumour patients everything will have changed since diagnosis. You may not be able to do what you once did. It is unlikely in the first year or two that you will be able to drive. You may have had to leave work, or change your career. You may struggle to hear or see or speak as you did. Watch and wait makes you feel like you can never plan ahead. As much as you may like to, and be urged to by your medical team, you can't simply go home and try to get back to normal.

My watch and wait periods have been defined by periods of mild depression, as well as feelings of being of no use to anyone. Between scans there doesn't seem to be time to start any new projects; what's the point if I'm going to be sick again in a few months' time? As a once successful small business owner, I found myself unable to continue in that way and went through various periods asking: Who am I? What am I for? What can I possibly become with this hanging over me?

It's extremely difficult to live in this way, and very hard for your friends and loved ones too when you reject their long term invites or continually answer 'I'm not sure', or 'As long as…'. Slowly you do get used to it, and if you have the confidence, you learn how to put your foot down and say: 'I'm sorry I just don't plan that far ahead'. Or, alternatively, you can stop saying 'no' and always say 'yes'. Everyone will understand if you are unable to attend a long planned event if your health takes a turn for the worse.

Brainstrust, a British brain tumour charity, is a specialist organisation that specialises in the emotional impacts of brain tumours among patients and their families. The charity recommends patients draw up a 'survivorship plan' tackling the biggest questions about their treatment, and the ongoing reality of living with a brain tumour. These form a great basis for final decisions with your oncologist before you are passed back to a watch and wait protocol. They will also help you to enlist help from charities if you don't feel you're getting the information or treatment you think you should be.

• Are you receiving the best possible treatment?

• Are you getting back to as normal a life as possible?

• Do you have easy access to the right information, tailored to your needs?

• Do you have financial security?

• Are you confident that any recurrence of cancer or any long term effects of treatment will be dealt with without delay and effectively?

• Are you confident you will be involved in any decision making, if you want to be?

• Do you have the confidence and skills to manage your condition yourself?

• Are your carers/loved ones included, if they want to be?[13]

> "I'm someone with quite a strong aversion to the typical support group, and I feel quite a violent reaction to the 'survivor' moniker and all attached to it. There's only so many times it can be handed out in your lifetime before it feels a little cruel if not patronising. I'm now in a very good place. I'm helping to build on the understanding of these diseases, I can (relatively) happily open myself up to that in the absence of a support group."
> Jack Webb

Duncan Weaver's first watch and wait period, from his initial diagnosis to his first surgery, lasted over two years. In that time, the real problem he faced was dealing with the epileptic seizures he was still having, and which various medications he was placed on – by doctors in the UK and in the Netherlands – had failed to bring under control.

After Duncan's first surgery and then radiotherapy, while his wife nursed their six week old baby, he developed a number of mobility problems. In particular, his right leg had become permanently numb meaning the couple had had to revise their plans and lifestyle to accommodate it.

But life went on, Duncan got used to his new disability, and the couple entered into a second long period of watch and wait. Much of this was taken up with Duncan trying to balance his newly acquired disability, the wonderful new addition to his family, and his and his wife's need to work to pay the bills.

Work was hard for Duncan. He'd still suffer from immense fatigue. The walk to the bus stop, previously taking just five minutes, turned into a 15 minute hobble. But work was important and he was determined not to give it up. He missed the banter with his colleagues, and working gave him a sense of purpose after feeling so useless since surgery and during his rehabilitation.

At home, they made a few adjustments to make life easier, and Duncan was determined he would still cycle despite his numb leg. After a few try out attempts, the couple settled on a *bakfiets*, a three wheeled bike the Dutch are famous for. It featured a large wooden box on the front which allowed Duncan to carry shopping, or occasionally his daughter, without the chance of toppling. Awkwardly strapped into the right pedal, Duncan gained back at least some of his freedom and independence.

And because his disability and fatigue meant he couldn't do many of the other things associated with looking after a toddler, that nursery run or taking little Tess to the park meant more to him than many of us can imagine.

Changes and challenges

"I LOST MY job through the early stages of my seizures and I can no longer insure myself in a self employed capacity. I can't drive or even confidently ride a bicycle, I can't practise or compete in the few physical pastimes I once enjoyed. To really galvanise my social life, I don't drink and I eat a restricted therapeutic diet. Any new relationships are started on uncertain footing to say the least. I know not all these problems are insurmountable, and some might even be considered a matter of perspective, but surgeries and treatments weigh as heavy on you as the tumour itself. It's hard to mobilise change when your focus is stunted and your energy is low."
Jack Webb

When you have been diagnosed with an anaplastic astrocytoma or a glioblastoma, it will quickly become clear that life as you knew it will never be the same again. Whether you choose to adopt the language and attitude of 'fighting' your brain tumour, or something more akin to being on a 'journey', your diagnosis is likely to influence and affect every aspect of your life, your sense of self, and your family and friends.

From not being certain if you can plan ahead, to having to break the news; from getting travel insurance to dealing with daily seizures or fatigue, brain tumours rarely let us patients rest on our laurels.

The British organisation The Brain Tumour Charity published a wide ranging study of patients in 2016 about their reported quality of life, called *Losing Myself*.[14] I'm pleased to credit this report for much of the material that follows. In *Losing Myself*, nine out of ten patients reported that their brain tumour had affected their emotional health, half said it had affected their finances, and half their memory. One in five experienced speech problems, one in four other cognitive problems.

As a patient myself, I have faced a host of physical and emotional obstacles over the last five years, many of which are reported by brain tumour patients of all sorts. There are a number of charities, Facebook groups, talkboards and other groups in which the same issues arise time and again. Thankfully charities and groups exist to help alleviate some of the frustrations, and answer some of the most difficult questions experienced by those of us with a life changing brain tumour.

My experience and those of others have shown that many friends, families and even doctors regard the major problem as the brain tumour itself. Get rid of it, and the problem has gone.

Unfortunately, life with a brain tumour doesn't

work that way. Anaplastic astrocytoma and glioblastoma bring along with them a huge number of changes and challenges which have to be dealt with, along with the tumour and the diagnosis.

This section aims to outline some of the main challenges a patient and their family will be facing, that are not directly medically connected. In a way, they may feel worse to the patient at times than having a life limiting illness.

"The tumour has changed our situation completely. With the breadwinner no longer bringing in any bread, we had to re-analyse where our future life would lead. I was the finance guy in a small company looking after budgeting, tax, legal, personnel: all the back office stuff. Now I cannot add up. It takes me a long time to write and read any important stuff. Physically I am well, probably stronger than I was before as I now do more outdoors work rather than working in front of a computer. Having had to move house has meant moving away from friends and much that goes with living in a small village. Being unable to drive has limited my ability to help my wife with simple things like going shopping."
Richard Stevens

Lack of direction

So your doctor has taken out the tumour as best they can. Your oncologist has hooked you up with treatment. Your scan will be in three months' time. After months of panic and fear, you're released back into the world and told to make the most of it. Reoccurance is certain. But no-one knows when.

What now?

There are plenty of anaplastic astrocytoma patients, and a number of glioblastoma patients, for whom treatment goes well. They know they may live another two, five, even 10 years, but what are they supposed to do with that time? The future is full of dissatisfaction and questions. Should I go back to my old job? Should I start/stop having babies? Should I get married? How will I earn a living? How will I afford the mortgage or rent?

There may be no satisfactory answer to these questions, but it is an ironic understatement to say you may lack direction in your life now you know where it is likely to go. For some patients, this is a release. They draw up a 'bucket list', travel the world seeing all the sights they promised they would, do all the wonderful things they hoped they would. They run a marathon and become an ambassador for a cancer charity. And good luck to them. Each has their own way of dealing with their prognosis.

But while the media and internet tend to hold such heroes in high esteem, most of us just aren't like that. At times my own diagnosis, and the lack of direction it has generated, has been paralysing. I've changed my mind about what I want to do for a job a thousand times, including doing no job at all. I've got into and out of new hobbies. I've wanted to travel the world. I've wanted to turn off the light and bury myself under a thick duvet. I've wanted to see long lost friends, make up for past wrongs; I've wanted to tell people what I really think about them, and be selfish with my time and money. For me there has been no consistency. No big project. And my family has had to face the ups and downs with me. They're the real heroes.

But it's okay to not know what you want to do. It's okay to sulk and cry and lock yourself away. It's okay to be depressed and despairing. What else do people expect you to be?

It is not my place to advise patients what to do for their own and their family's wellbeing. However, there are professionals who you may wish to consult if you want to try to shape the rest of your life. You may not be able to plan for the long term, but even short term goals may help make you feel more solid, and your family more secure.

You can access counselling, group therapy, cognitive behavioural therapy, mediation or whatever you think might work. You can also become part of the 'brain tumour community' posting your own questions – and your own answers – on Facebook pages, sharing and advising and gaining strength when you need it.

No-one expects you to have a smile on your face, or to climb Mount Everest – unless you want to. People want to support you, and when you think you know what you might want to do, let them know and you'll be surprised by how helpful people can be.

Fatigue

Tiredness is probably the most talked about subject, next to treatment, on brain tumour talkboards and Facebook groups. It seems everyone with a brain tumour experiences chronic fatigue, and regularly. And no surprise: both brain tumours, and medication for seizures and swelling, are key causes of incredible, almost indescribable fatigue. In *Losing Myself*, three in five respondents reported fatigue as a significant symptom of their brain tumour. More than 40 percent of those said they were severely affected by it.

Fatigue is not just tiredness. I like to think of tiredness as a comfortable droopy eyed, ready-for-bed sleepiness you get at the end of the day. Everyone gets tired. Fatigue is something else entirely. It is a heaviness that encompasses your whole body and feels like it is physically preventing you from doing things or even thinking straight. You find yourself pulling your body up stairs. It is an effort to put one foot in front of another. Just the idea of doing work (whether looking after an infant, working at a computer, or pushing around a vacuum cleaner) is tiring itself, let alone carrying it out.

I have suffered fatigue at times ever since I took my first anti-seizure medication, in 2012. And during a year of cancer treatment, I've suffered fatigue so severe I simply have not been able to function. On the worst days, if I could get out of bed at all, I would manage breakfast before going back to bed to sleep for two or three hours. I'd then sleep again in the afternoon. This wasn't a choice or laziness, I just could not do anything but go to sleep.

Bear in mind that I consider myself extremely fit, and before diagnosis was a racing cyclist: this fatigue has hit me extremely hard. It's eaten into my very sense of self – the active, quick and agile man I once was feels like he has been replaced by a slow, lumpy drag of wet clay.

One not very helpful commentator on my blog, after I'd written about this fatigue, told me I was depressed, not tired. I needed to get out more. Take exercise. This poster clearly had never experienced serious fatigue, nor paid attention to the rest of my blog where I wrote regularly about my being an active cyclist. The fatigue may have caused me to be frustrated, even sad, but it was not depression. I know what depression feels like, and I know a killer way to ease it when I can is to take some exercise. But fatigue is sheer, body knackeredness. Your muscles and skin feel like they're hanging from your creaking bones. I could barely climb on a bike, let alone go out for a cycle.

As The Brain Tumour Charity's *Losing Myself* report comments: "Many people living with a brain tumour find they can no longer take part in leisure activities, with seven in 10 people in this study telling us they had given up or reduced their participation in sport or exercise. Previously nurtured skills or hobbies may become impossible to pursue due to loss of physical function or concentration, and pain or fatigue."

Clinicians suggest those who suffer extreme fatigue do some regular, light exercise to ease the symptoms. Where possible, walking the dog, or the kids to school, or just doing the shopping, count as light exercise. Achieving just that is what patients should be aiming for, not a spin class or a half marathon. Indeed, my experience is that pushing myself too hard when I'm suffering fatigue makes the tiredness even worse the next day.

More important even than regular light exercise, I'd argue – and so would many brain tumour support groups – is to go easy on yourself. It's okay to be fatigued. It is a real symptom of your condition, just as significant as the surgery scar on your head.

When my wife and I decided that it was okay for me to be fatigued and to take sleep breaks most days –

to not feel guilty – it made a considerable difference to my mental health and wellbeing (and hers too). My children say they've never known me not to sleep during the day. My fatigue is normal to them, so it should be normal to me. Guilt comes part and parcel of brain tumours in so many ways. Don't let fatigue contribute to it.

Nausea

Another symptom of brain tumours – whether it comes from the tumour itself and from anti-seizure drugs (which is frequent), or chemotherapy (which is practically guaranteed) – is feeling sick. Depending on where your tumour is located, it has the potential to affect your balance, reactions, eyesight, hearing and hormone producing glands, all of which can create nausea. But severe headaches, caused by pressure in the skull created by a brain tumour, can also generate nausea and vomiting.

In either case, once your tumour has been identified, you are likely to be placed on anti-sickness medication. You may also be given steroids such as dexamethasone. Unfortunately, both of these medicines have their own side effects. For antiemetics, these include irritability, constipation and fatigue, while steroids can lead to poor sleep, increased appetite and weight gain.

In my experience, asking to take the minimum of both drug types while balancing that against their side effects, and the treatment effect they have, has been the way forward. During radiotherapy, I regularly took anti-sickness medication, but it made me so constipated that I decided I'd prefer to feel slightly sick most of the time than experience long, painful periods on the toilet.

I fought the nausea with chewing gum and strongly flavoured sweets.

As a cyclist I'm practically paranoid about my weight, but so far have been able to avoid taking too many steroids (though more than would allow me to participate in the *Tour de France*, that's for sure). If a larger dose of steroids was proposed in the future, my own vanity might prevent me from taking them until I really had no choice.

At the end of the day, your doctors will always seek to balance the medication you need with the side effects you experience. They will also take into account your own personal preferences. They come from an attitude of doing the least possible harm to you, your body and your mental health. In all but very specific circumstances you have a right to refuse any treatment, and to ask for a second opinion.

Personality change

> "I am a lot more frustrated when I cannot do what I used to be able to do. I am a lot more easily roused. I have been known to swear more than I used to; I tend to be rather a polite chap most of the time. I lose my temper much more quickly than I used to. This whole situation is very, very frustrating."
> Richard Stevens

When I began seeing my neurologist regularly, he would address me but also ask my wife a series of questions: Had she noticed any changes in me or the way I behaved? Was I acting normally, the way I did before? It turned out, he told us, that it was likely she would notice any behavioural change before I did.

Brain tumours, if they grow in particular parts of the brain, can be responsible for significant personality change, and usually for the worse. Patients can become irritable, even angry, selfish and depressed. These are not just emotional responses to the tumour, but a physiological symptom of pressure build up in particular parts of the brain. Tumours in the frontal lobe are particularly known for causing personality change, because that is where emotional processing takes place in the brain. Tumours on or close to the pituitary gland, which controls hormone release, can change moods.

In *Losing Myself*, 28 percent of people diagnosed with a brain tumour reported experiencing some form of personality change. Personally, as my tumour has progressed and my treatment too, I'll admit to losing my temper more easily, being less patient with my children than I'd like to be, and generally just finding the world too much. Thankfully, in my case, this has not resulted in violence. But I can easily see how it can and does tip over into that among some patients. Some families report their once docile and warm hearted loved one becoming a different person at times, or even permanently, as a result of their brain tumour and treatment.

Anxiety, depression, anger, short temper, mood swings, aggression, inability to measure feelings, loss of inhibitions, memory problems and emotional blankness, they're all possible. Even probable.

Support groups – for patients, and for loved ones – are very important here, because behaviour change can become unmanageable at times. It's hard not to lay blame or compare the patient to 'the old you' when tempers are frayed and stress is high, and of course physical and verbal violence is never acceptable.

But it is important for patients and families to seek and receive support when it feels like things are getting out of hand. Carers are just as important as patients, so everyone needs to ensure they and the patient are comfortable and safe.

Reading self help books on anger and anxiety – as I have done, where previously I'd never have given it a second thought – joining a counselling group, seeing a psychotherapist, and meditation and mindfulness exercises, all are reported to help ease tension and head off emotional explosions. Brain tumour charities and relationship counselling services often have very good helplines to support people in emotional crisis, whether a patient or family member.

Doctors may also be able to prescribe anti-anxiety medication and anti-depressants, as well as steroids to reduce swelling that is putting pressure on emotion governing areas of the brain. For particularly serious personality disorders, you may be able to get an appointment with a neuropsychologist or psychiatrist. They specialise in the effects of brain disease on mental abilities and behaviour.

Loved ones may have to stretch their tolerance to breaking point to demonstrate to the patient they are still loved, despite their behaviour, and that they want to work with them to manage their emotional problems. At the end of the day, brain tumours affect personal relationships, including even the closest of marriages. Their impact stretches far beyond the medical, and all involved need to be aware of the impact they can have immediately and as the disease progresses.

The Brain Tumour Charity publishes a very useful factsheet, that can be accessed free online.[15]

> "One thing I wish I'd known is to be prepared for the personality changes, especially aggression and difficult behaviour. Nobody is told to expect this, let alone how to handle it or seek support. This is a job you can only do well if you totally love the person, because no-one else would be able to handle those demands."
> Joanna Waters, sister to Sue Rossides

Relationship problems

Closely related to behaviour change is the pressure created in personal relationships between patients and their partners, families, loved ones and friends. According to *Losing Myself*, two in three respondents said the tumour had impacted on their relationship with their partner. Three quarters reported the disease affecting their physical intimacy. Family members report loved ones becoming introverted and uninterested; they can be hard work to care for, demanding and unsympathetic.

There is a very real need for couples and families to take professional advice and counselling to help maintain relationships, if that is what is wanted. It sounds like a cliché, but admitting there is a problem is likely to be the hardest but most significant step.

For some it will be too much, but others will be determined to overcome the barriers that grow between them as the disease progresses.

As *Losing Myself* cites: "Studies show that it is the personality and cognitive effects of brain tumours that place most strain on relationships, particularly where they cause behaviour change, and that interventions to manage challenging behaviour and increase caregiver knowledge can make a positive difference."[16]

Pain

It is well known that the brain itself has no pain receptors, and that if you could gently prod your brain with your finger you would not feel a thing. Unfortunately, the brain is surrounded by bone, tissue, skin and muscles, all of which have nerves and can hurt very much. Indeed, massive unbearable migraine headaches, most often caused by pressure in the skull, are one of the symptoms that send brain tumour patients to accident and emergency departments.

Losing Myself reports that nearly half of all brain tumour patients said they lived with constant pain: "The degree of pain and incapacity endured as a result of chronic headaches, migraine and accompanying nausea can be completely debilitating, confining people to bed to 'sleep it off' or to recover from drowsiness caused by strong pain relief. One participant described constant head pain: 'I go to bed with a headache and wake with one'; another reported having migraines '24/7'." Reports of missing out on family life as a consequence of chronic pain were common, it said.

Head pain is just the beginning. Those who find themselves wheelchair users, temporarily or permanently bed bound, or more susceptible to falls may have the pain of bed sores, grazes and broken bones to deal with too.

So the idea that brain tumours are pain free is a myth, and in some cases brain pressure thanks to a tumour can be so painful that morphine or other high dose painkiller drugs are needed. Towards the end of life, when nothing else can be done to release pressure or prevent growth, many patients are medicated to go into a 'morphine coma', freeing them of pain for short or longer periods. Sometimes they never wake up which, with consent, might be the unspoken intention.

If your own doctor or oncologist is unable to help you with your pain, many hospitals and health centres – particularly those with cancer centres – have pain management clinics. It is well worth trying to book an appointment with the consultants there, as they will be specialists in all types of pain, and the drugs, exercises and strategies that work best.

The American Brain Tumor Association has a factsheet on managing pain, particularly severe headaches relating to your tumour. It suggests patients keep a headache or pain journal, so that you can provide an accurate, consistent and comparable record to doctors when you report your symptoms. The charity says it is not unusual for symptoms to change over time, and those changes can be significant, so it is essential to keep track.[17]

Alcohol

You should not drink any alcohol during chemotherapy treatment, as it will clash with your drugs. It is inadvisable to take alcohol with anti-seizure medication too, though each type of medication will have its own advisory information. You should read the instructions carefully.

It is likely that you will have reduced or cut out alcohol from your diet altogether, thanks to your brain tumour. For some, this is no problem but others may have previously been dependent on alcohol, physically or as a social lubricant. It's certainly difficult to meet friends who are all drinking and to order a lemonade. We all need to feel part of a social group, and for good or ill those of us who are part of groups in which drink plays a role may find ourselves excluded, self censored, or merely put off from socialising.

Oh, for the taste of a good red wine or a chilled glass of real Guinness in an Irish pub! I genuinely miss the taste of alcohol, particularly my favourite good English ales. When I was first diagnosed, I continued to drink occasionally. Indeed, I perhaps depended on a drink to take away some of the stress of what my family was going through. But mixed with my anti-seizure medication, I found that I would get heavier hangovers than before, and they lasted longer. In the end, I decided that I preferred to feel well when I could, than to sacrifice good mornings when I could be socialising, playing with my kids or cycling.

In social circles – among cycling buddies, friends, and even family – it has been hard becoming known as a non-drinker, as if I'm spoiling the party. But these are selfish thoughts. Most of the time, others don't even notice you're not drinking because they're too busy behind their own glass.

Language confusion

The brain is, of course, responsible for governing language, both the understanding and processing of what is said to you, and what you say and express to others.

When brain tumours emerge in the language and speech processing areas of the brain, very common in glioma tumours like astrocytoma and glioblastoma, it is likely the patient may have language processing problems.

The impact is wide ranging. It can be minimal, such as the inability to put words together during a short lived partial focal seizure, or the temporary inability to name particular objects. I experience both of these on a regular basis. During a seizure, I know what I'm trying to say, but what comes out of my mouth is nonsense and garbled. This is known as asphasia. At other times, I just can't find the right word for everyday objects, and end up asking my kids to get the milk from the 'big cold thing'. This is called dysphasia. Forgetting the name of places and people, or just having them on the tip of my tongue, can sometimes be another challenge.

As the *Losing Myself* report says: "One in five people reported having speech problems as a result of their brain tumour. People told us of the embarrassment and anxiety that comes from living with aphasia, or speech disorders. One female participant explained that she felt she could never say what she meant: 'I am never quick enough and can often throw in the wrong word, which is totally irrelevant in a sentence'."

For others, language problems are more severe. Brain tumour patients may, at times, be unable to process what is being said to them, or what they are reading and hearing. Nor are they able to communicate in ways in which they once could. When language problems start to become more severe, it is worth asking for a referral to a speech and language therapist who may be able to set up a programme of relearning ways to communicate so the patient does not become completely isolated.

The fantastic materials already produced for dementia and Alzheimer's patients, as well as for those with learning difficulties, can be particularly useful here. They're tried and tested, and like sign language for deaf people, are becoming recognised and consistent around the world. Many public bodies now produce *easy-read* versions of their publications, with simple words and lots of pictures, which may assist brain tumour patients with understanding and expressing themselves if their own speech and writing is beginning to fail. The emphasis of *easy-read* materials is on enabling people to continue living their lives independently, not on spoon feeding patients as if they were babies who have lost their capacity to think.

Driving

In the UK, this is by far the most popular subject for complaint and concern among brain tumour patients. Comments on Facebook support groups for brain tumour patients run to page after page, complaining about not being able to drive, and the battle to get driving licences back.

It is no exaggeration to state that patients are driven to distraction and despair by their sudden inability to drive, and an apparent uphill struggle to be re-granted the right to drive later on in their brain tumour journey. The Brain Tumour Charity's helpline for patients reports it as one of the most frequently arising issues. *Losing Myself* says of one respondent: "Passionate about the freedom driving gives her, she has described losing her licence as the single most emotionally damaging aspect of her condition, making her reliant on others to go about her daily life."[18]

Under UK legislation, any type of brain tumour diagnosis will see a patient banned from driving for at least three months, probably far more. The exact conditions under which someone can get their driving license back will always vary according to their tumour type, and their seizure pattern. Under current legislation, those who have had an epileptic fit or seizure must be seizure free for at least a year before they can drive again. Anyone who undergoes treatment such as surgery, radiotherapy or chemotherapy for a brain tumour must wait for two years after treatment is complete before being able to get back behind the wheel. And if the patient has a new seizure or a new treatment, the clock is reset. Moreover, the driving authorities in the UK have been heavily criticised by patients, charities and even a Parliamentary committee for making random and inconsistent decisions about individuals' ability to drive when they have a brain tumour.

> "Before this time I was very much a petrol
> head. Now I am reliant on lifts everywhere and
> have lost my travel independence. Yes, it's
> frustrating, but that's secondary to staying
> alive. Luckily I work a lot from home, and even
> luckier I spend more time with my wife who
> drives me everywhere. It may be rare but we
> really do enjoy each other's company. Having a
> disabled railcard has proven very useful."
> Graham Dunnett

In the US, ability to drive with or after a brain tumour and treatment are assessed and governed on a state by state basis.

Let me be clear. Though we've all got used to doing it, driving a car, motorcycle or even bigger vehicle is a complex task. Patients diagnosed with a brain tumour are at a higher accident risk, because of the risk of seizures, memory lapses and cognitive dysfunctions. It is essential that governments account for these, and they rightly impose restrictions on those of us with brain tumours and seizures, however frustrating.

But it doesn't stop it from being frustrating – for the patient, and for loved ones. In my case, I felt immediately redundant after having my driving licence taken away. I lived in the countryside in England, and could no longer drive even to the nearest shop. I was lucky to work from home and to be a cyclist, but I couldn't take my children to the park or for a swim without having to plan bus routes. Even trips to the hospital had to be made by bicycle or bus, or else my wife would have to take time out from work to transport me.

Eventually, when the prospect of my driving again became impossible to imagine, we had to move home. We ended up in a small town, on a mainline train into a major city, with good transport connections. The isolation had made it impossible to continue to live where we were.

The inability to drive is paralysing for brain tumour patients, and a heavy burden on others to provide lifts – not only to hospital and appointments, but to just get on with life. Western society has simply become so reliant on our cars. It's no surprise that feelings of helplessness, loss, even grief and depression quickly follow. In some cases, the ability to drive is very much part of our sense of self. Driving is what adults do, and there's a feeling of dropping our kids off at school or at a friend's house as something like a right. Brain tumour patients are suddenly robbed of these simple indicators of our maturity.

It's simply another case of a diagnosis of brain tumour being far greater than the life limiting disease itself, but impacting on every aspect of a patient's life.

Work

> "I used to be a flight attendant; I really loved my job, it was my dream. Sadly, I wasn't able to pursue my career following my diagnosis. I was devastated. Thankfully, the airline that I worked for was very supportive – offering me a switch to ground duties and being patient and understanding with me. My brain cancer diagnosis completely changed my work life. Some days I feel as though I have been cheated out of so many adventures and work opportunities that I would have had as a crew member, but then I remind myself that I'm lucky to be alive. That helps to put things into perspective."
> Calum Wright

All of us want to feel productive, whether in a paid job, in a voluntary position, in the home or elsewhere. Brain tumours can swing a wrecking ball through our ability to do any kind of work, destroying not only our incomes, but our very sense of purpose.

If you have an employer, they may be impatient to find out what you are planning to do. When will you return to work? Should they recruit to replace you? Perhaps they have to stop your sick pay, and you might have to go into a social benefits system.

Legislation is obviously different across the world regarding illness, disability and work. Those who are employed should consult their own HR departments, charities and citizens advice organisations to see what their illness and retirement rights are.

The *Losing Myself* report reports that 28 percent of all brain tumour patients had to give up work entirely as a result of their illness, and one in five had had to reduce their working hours. For anaplastic astrocytoma and glioblastoma patients, I imagine the proportions will be far higher. Three in four respondents said their own and/or their partner's working life had also been affected, and half said they had been hit financially as a result of their tumour. "Working created my identity and that has gone, leaving me empty and invaluable," reported one 60 year old man with a high grade tumour.

The results of losing work of any kind are many fold, including losing a sense of self and purpose, depression and financial difficulties. The problems are too complex to deal with here, but charities and helplines are well placed to advise you on your specific circumstances, any benefits you may be entitled to and any extra help you may be able to get to accommodate your health problems regarding your work.

In my experience, even before treatment I found I could not work consistently and reliably as a writer and editorial consultant. During treatment, fatigue was so intense, I was unable to complete projects on time, and totally lost my motivation to look for freelance work. I wasn't even sure I could complete anything that came my way. The result was depression.

Encouraged by my wife, I looked into a voluntary opportunity that would keep me physically and mentally active while fatigue, illness and treatment held me back. I began working at a workshop that refurbished bicycles, bringing old rusted wrecks back to life for sale in charity shops. Not only did the opportunity come with no obligations to do a certain number of hours at a certain time, meaning I could rest when I needed to, but I learned new skills that complemented one of my key passions. Many patients may not be able or motivated to search out other opportunities to 'work' or reignite passion in anything after what they have been through. I do consider myself lucky.

"We had to move as I had little or no income. My employer deliberately did not pay me my monthly salary and I had to point out that that was illegal before I received the money. I had a mortgage to pay. That was not all that was owed to me and I had to take her to court before we reached an agreement. I had not intended to retire for a long time. Any planning went straight out of the window."
Richard Stevens

"My employer knows that I have had (and still have) problems that make my work very hard. I am a director that manages a team of support engineers. I set up the UK office, increased the staff here and work life was great. Then, I had my seizures – the start of two years of brain tumour and work problems. My employer knows what I am like, and how days and weeks and months vary. They treat me now exactly the same as they always have. But my role has been simplified, and I learned that as my technical and mental capacities

were falling away, my daily work was made non-critical. A company allowing a brain tumour employee to work this way must surely be unique."
Graham Dunnett

Travel and other insurances

If you have been diagnosed with a life limiting brain tumour, the simple truth is that you will not be given life insurance by any provider. You're simply not a good bet for them, as you or your loved ones are pretty much bound to need to make a claim at some point.

You may have been smart enough (some would say lucky), as I was, to take out critical illness insurance before you were diagnosed – though I did cancel one of my two policies just a few months before going to the doctors for the first time. Being able to pay of our mortgage helped us to take some time off work, to come to terms with what had happened. Though the money could not last forever. If you have recently been diagnosed and do not have a life insurance policy – do check whether there's a policy attached to your job or mortgage – you may be in an especially vulnerable position. In the very likely circumstance that your diagnosis affects your ability to work, you may find yourself on a pretty strict budget, perhaps dependent on state benefits, charity handouts, and generous friends and family.

Holidays may be the last thing on your mind if you have been recently diagnosed, but once the shock and initial treatment are over, you may find a break away is exactly what you and your family need. You may be accustomed to easily getting travel insurance, to cover your baggage, cancellation, repatriation and medical expenses for while you are away, should things go wrong. Unfortunately, a malignant brain tumour sets you apart.

In many cases, brain tumour patients find themselves unable to get insurance at all, or the premiums are so steep that they cost almost as much as the holiday itself. I have not been able to get travel insurance via an online search engine. I just don't fit their criteria, and the moment you tick serious medical condition, you're asked to call the insurance provider directly, essentially to be told you can't be covered, or that it'll cost you so much you might as well not bother.

This is frustrating because at the time when you most need and want to take a holiday – after all, in the worst case it may be your last with your family – you can't get the reassurance that you'll be looked after if anything goes wrong.

In the UK, successive governments are starting to wake up to this contradiction. Some specialist insurance providers are beginning to offer very limited policies, and brain tumour and cancer charities, as well as talkboards and support groups, will be able to share their own experiences and recommendations.

Depression

> "Sue's depression continued to deepen. I rang her doctor and he recommended Seroxat (an anti-depressant). This was like a magic pill, it worked instantly. But then she started to retreat into her own little world. Her memory gradually faded until she reached the point where she had no understanding of what had

happened to her or why she was bedridden. I very much doubted if she would reach her birthday. She did, but I had to tell her repeatedly throughout the day. Tragically, she snapped out of it at the end of the day and said, 'I don't want to be like this forever'. Thankfully, she showed no memory of this the next day and in fact this was the last time she showed any understanding."

Joanna Waters, sister of Sue Rossides

I've mentioned depression a number of times in both side effects and life challenges of a brain tumour diagnosis, and its power should not be underestimated. Many brain tumour patients feel they have, often suddenly, had everything taken away from them. Their future life, their hopes and ambitions, their work, their ability to drive, their personal relationships. What is there to be happy about?

But depression isn't just a lack of happiness. It features a very real despair that things can't and won't get better; that perhaps you don't deserve for them to get better; a sense of worthlessness and burden. Just getting out of bed is hard work, no matter how many people try to visit with a smile, or want to see you, or tell you all the positive things going on in your life. The famous 'black dog' will sit on your shoulders, bringing you down, even on the brightest days.

Depression is a mental illness. Some of us are more susceptible to it than others, but it would be rare for a brain tumour patient not to feel low at least some of the time. Most of us know the black dog is at our heels much of the time, if not wholly consuming us.

Thankfully, no-one should blame you for feeling

low after a brain tumour diagnosis. This gives you a platform to start to get better. The first step is to admit that you are depressed, and the second is to understand that you will not get better without help. With depression, often the last thing you will want to do is to talk about it. But if you can reach out far enough to call a helpline or the doctor, or to take the hand of a parent, sibling or close friend, and tell them you need some help, it will hopefully start the ball rolling.

Ideally, you'll be able to establish regular talking sessions, counselling or cognitive behavioural therapy, which are proven ways to lift you out of the doldrums. You'll be able to talk and write about your problems, including your most wild and intimate self criticisms and fears, without judgement. You'll lighten the burden, and your counsellor will help you to see the brighter side of things where possible.

In my experience, three things have been of significant help. First, cliché though it is, is the loving support of my partner. Though she does not have previous experience of depression, she has come to understand the importance and reality of it in my life. She has been able to respond, providing me with space and time to talk, and pointed me towards professional help when I've needed it.

That professional help is the second relieving factor. I have taken counselling where I've been able to talk about my feelings, unearthing deep rooted problems that have nothing to do with my illness, but which have been brought into relief by it. When things are at their lowest point, I have money set aside for professional counselling because I know it works for me.

Finally, the slow but general acceptance, at least in

the West, of depression as a real mental illness, and one that occurs naturally, has made a difference to me. Today, you can tell a friend that you are feeling depressed and need some space, and most are sympathetic. You can access online materials, and schoolchildren are even taught about depression and mental wellbeing. One YouTube video in particular helped both me and my wife understand the nature of depression, normalising it for both of us.[19] The video written and illustrated by Matthew Johnstone, *I had a black dog, and his name was depression,* has now become a bestselling picture book, with another book published in the series aimed at carers. It is not brain tumour specific, but many of the themes will be familiar.

Of course, doctors can also prescribe medicines for anxiety and depression, and these can be very effective indeed. You must consult with your medical team before beginning, or reinstating, any anti-depressant regime, because there is a significant risk that those drugs will interact negatively with any radiation, chemotherapy and anti-seizure medication you may be taking.

Guilt

Guilt can be another life challenge, especially for those who are living relatively normal lives after being given a long watch and wait period. The realisation that life will never the be the same again is a difficult part of having an ultimately life limiting brain tumour. However hard you try, it is impossible to put your old life back together even if your prognosis appears relatively good.

Nevertheless, friends might presume that you are better or well again. Life can go on, because you're out of danger. You know this is far from the truth. It's hard to watch others get on with their lives, wiping their brow, thanking lady luck or whoever for your favourable outcome, and assuming everything is now okay. After the initial fuss when you are first diagnosed, or during and after your treatment, friends and loved ones will naturally drop away to get on with their lives.

You may even feel guilty – as I did – for not dying. For causing such a fuss without following up on the promise. Of course, nobody really feels this way about your illness. Everyone is glad you've made it through so far, but none of us can remain in panic all of the time. Rest assured your friends and loved ones will return if things become urgent again.

Another aspect of guilt you may feel is that there's every chance you're still having seizures, or headaches, and you will almost certainly be seriously fatigued from the drugs you have to take. You may feel guilty about not being able to help with the kids, to cook for yourself, to do your share of the housework. As a 40 year old man and a father of three, having to sleep for an hour or more some days since diagnosis has generated enormous guilt. My wife has had to take care of the children, or I've left them to play by themselves. Surely, when my life is ultimately limited, I should be spending every second I can with them? But sometimes I'm just too tired.

Finally, and this is perhaps the worst of it, watch and wait can generate feelings of guilt relating to your own luck in having a tumour that is responding to treatment. As you become a patient, and a member of the brain tumour community, you might meet other people with brain tumours like yours. If your own tumour is responding well, it is likely you will get to know others whose journey is not running so smoothly. I have felt this acutely, as new friends I have made since diagnosis have passed away. Closely married to my grief for the loss of friends is the guilt that I'm still alive. That my family have, so far, been spared the pain I can see their loved ones experiencing.

It is not easy to experience these mental difficulties, alongside the physical difficulties a brain tumour might produce. More significantly, you might find there is far less support for those experiencing depression, anxiety and guilt, than for those facing physical difficulties – particularly outside of the hospital or clinical setting. This is where charities can be invaluable, as well as Facebook and other social media groups for brain tumour patients. They know what you are going through, they can offer encouragement and will recommend sources of support. My own book, *Brain Tumours: Living Low Grade*, has longer sections on living longer with a brain tumour, particularly my own and others' experience of watch and wait, and the emotions it can generate.

> "I was driven to research all I could. For every awful loss I had to find a survivor. I had also to be prepared to help George with any questions he may want to ask. I felt very alone in a family situation when everyone was thinking it was all over and recovery would be 100 percent. I think I felt differently from the outset. I found the American Brain Tumor Association a lifeline and various UK websites, and I read many blogs and connected on Facebook with others facing similar situations."
> Jane Cooke, mother of George

Seizures

Seizures are another of the biggest issues for brain tumour patients, because they can be a weekly or even daily reminder of the tumour, and a limitation on living life to the full.[20]

Though seizures are most frequently reported in lower grade brain tumours, some 40 to 60 percent of glioblastoma patients report some kind of seizure.[21] Of those with high grade tumours, those that report seizures tend to have smaller tumours.[22]

Seizures might be the reason they came to a doctor in the first place, or they may be something that develops after diagnosis. An understanding of how the brain works explains why brain tumours are likely to cause seizures. The brain is comprised of billions of neurons, which are brain cells that process and transmit information between each other as electrical pulses. In most brains, the transmissions fire off in a relatively straightforward pattern, with only occasional misfires. But when neurons are disrupted, causing irregular firing of electrical signals, it can cause a seizure.

In some brain tumours, the neurological disturbance can remain quite localised. This causes partial, or focal, seizures. Only parts or single functions of the body might be affected, for a short time, and you'll remain conscious and remember the seizure afterwards.

In other brain tumours, the neurological disturbance might spread across the whole brain, creating a massive disturbance in all areas. This type of seizure most often leads to tonic clonic (formerly known as *grand mal*) or generalised seizures, under which patients become unconscious. It is these seizures we most often associate with epilepsy, or fitting on the ground.

Brain tumour patients can experience either or both types of seizures. Or, of course, no seizures at all.

Partial/simple seizures

These are named not because they affect part of your body, but because the neurological disturbance in the brain is localised. They are also known as focal seizures. They might entail one or more of the following:

- Involuntary movement of limbs, neck muscles
- Twitches, strangeness in arms, hands, feet
- Inability to speak or muddled language
- Palsy: paralysis or tremors in muscles, such as those controlling the mouth and face
- Absence or staring into space, feeling or acting 'lost' or disconnected
- *Déjà vu*
- Lip smacking, pulling at clothing
- Strange taste or hearing sensations.

Sometimes localised seizures can become more widespread across the brain, and turn into tonic clonic seizures.

Tonic clonic seizures

These are the seizures we most often associate with epilepsy, though there are actually more than 40 different types.[23] Typically, they go through three phases:

• Tonic: The patient will suddenly stiffen and fall to the ground, immediately followed by the stiffening of their muscles, their back arched. There may be some trouble breathing, as the chest contracts. The tonic phase is unlikely to last more than a minute.

• Clonic: Very quickly, the patient will move to this phase. Muscles will spasm and jerk quickly, then the fitting will gradually slow down until ceasing altogether, often concluding with a deep sigh. The clonic phase usually lasts around two minutes.

The tonic and clonic aspects of the seizure can take anything up to five minutes. Any longer, or if seizures occur one after the other, without recovery, you should seek medical assistance.

• Recovery: The patient may not come out of unconsciousness right away. They may wake confused, scared and fatigued and require support to understand what has happened as they come round.

If you find yourself vulnerable to any kind of seizure as a result of your tumour, it is suggested you consult your doctors on how you, your family and others should react, as well as when emergency services should be called.

Whether partial or generalised, many of those who have seizures report experiencing a strange feeling a minute to 30 seconds before one begins.

This is known as an 'aura', and can include tingling, *déjà vu*, 'buffering' in the brain or a strange taste. But some receive no warning at all.

Anti-seizure medication
After you have been diagnosed with a brain tumour, it is very likely that you will be given anti-

seizure medication. For most patients, you will remain on some kind of anti-seizure drugs for the rest of your life. The drugs aim to maintain balance in neurological activity in the brain, as if wrapping it in cotton wool to dampen down abnormal electrical surges.

If you have received surgery, the scarring and intervention of the surgery itself can be a cause of seizures. Radiation and chemotherapy treatments can also cause seizures, as brain tumours grow, contract, or the brain is affected by swelling.

Treatment and surgery

The removal or reduction in size of your brain tumour may affect the types and regularity of the seizures you have. Though initially surgery may lead to more frequent seizures, the hope would be an eventual reduction in seizures as the tumour becomes smaller.

Seizures can also have particular triggers. For example, I can sometimes prompt a seizure if my body temperature is high. I've had one in a sauna and often have them when I am doing intensive exercise. Others find fatigue, stress or alcohol can bring them on.

If you do not currently have seizures, you may develop them. Or the seizures you currently have might change in their intensity, frequency or type. The brain is a complex piece of machinery, much of it far from understood by even the most expert neurologists. It's worth noting that an increase in seizures, or their intensity, is not necessarily an indication that a tumour has regrown or intensified – though it certainly can be.

It is worth keeping a diary of seizures, their type and intensity, to share with your doctors, so they can consider your seizure patterns, anti-epileptic drugs, MRI scans and treatments in the round.

Lack of exercise and lack of motivation so often go together. James Campling had been a corporal in the Aeromedical Evacuation Squadron in the Royal Air Force (RAF). When he was diagnosed, he was at the peak of fitness. Even though, as a nurse, he was in a non-combat role, he had to drill, exercise and push his body to the limits just to do his job. His annual fitness test was one of the most gruelling of the year.

So the fatigue and mental draining that came with his brain tumour diagnosis, and the intense treatment that followed, hit him hard. He thought it would be a quick recovery, but all of a sudden his body just had nothing. With everything that had happened, he couldn't motivate himself to go for anything more than a short walk, perhaps a bike ride. The radiotherapy in particular sapped him of his energy.

Worst thing was, it was such a departure from what he had been doing before. He quickly fell out of step with his fitter friends and colleagues. Their social and military life had been based around fitness; now he didn't fit in. Everything had changed. His work was sympathetic, but the RAF could only pay him sick leave for so long. No longer able to work as a frontline nurse, James was offered an office job pushing paper around. There would be no patient contact, no contact with his fellow medics, he'd lose out on a lot.

There were a lot of positives to working for the RAF – a generous pension, a commitment to keeping him working – but they were 100 percent outweighed by the negatives. He couldn't pursue his old career. He couldn't get promoted.

And there was something else. Something he tried not to think about too much, but which niggled him.

He was 28 years old, and any hope of starting a family was ebbing away. In the space of a few months, he felt he'd lost everything. There was only one thing for it. To plan for more travelling.

Just weeks after an MRI following his chemotherapy and radiotherapy showed no new tumour, James booked a ticket. This time to Antarctica.

Diet

Can eating a specific diet, or drinking certain drinks or other substances, improve your chances of getting through treatment better, slow down your tumour's growth, or even cure your cancer altogether?

I do not seek to be controversial here, so I withhold personal judgement except to say I am skeptical of the claims made by many 'cancer gurus' about supposed miracle cures, such as specific diets or smoothies. The science simply does not bear them out.

The charity Cancer Research UK, backed by the UK's National Health Service, says: "the term 'superfood' is really just a marketing tool, with little scientific basis. It's certainly true that a healthy, balanced and varied diet can help to reduce the risk of cancer but it is unlikely that any single food will make a major difference on its own."

The Brain Tumour Charity in the UK says: "A healthy diet is associated with numerous general health benefits, including reducing the risk of other medical conditions such as diabetes, heart disease, as well as some types of cancer. Adopting a healthier diet after being diagnosed with a brain tumour could benefit you in the following ways: keeping up your strength and energy; maintaining your weight and your body's store of nutrients; lowering your risk of infection; aiding the healing and recovery process..."

"While the overall benefits of following a healthy diet have always been stressed by healthcare professionals, there is an ongoing discussion and a need for ongoing research about the potential role of diet and nutrition in the treatment of brain tumours."[24]

The American Brain Tumor Association (ABTA) has a very good webinar on brain tumours and nutrition, repeating the notion that general good healthy living and balanced eating will help patients recover from treatment and manage symptoms. But that there is no magical food or ingredient known to prevent, cause or cure brain tumours. It does note that brain tumours could change a patient's relationship with food, as treatment will change both the taste and enjoyment of food, as well as their appetite.

The charity has some great advice on how thinking about diet and cooking can ease symptoms and encourage appetite. It suggests using strong flavours to combat nausea, eating little and often, as well as avoiding greasy, high fat foods. It advises eating high fibre foods to ease constipation.

ABTA says that food supplements have not been proven to improve outcomes for brain tumour outcomes. There's no way to guarantee what's in a supplement you're taking, because they don't have to be approved by the Federal Drugs Administration (FDA), though the FDA can remove it from sale if found to be unsafe. ABTA warns that natural supplements can negatively interact with chemotherapy drugs, so patients should consult very carefully with their oncologist before taking anything.[25]

Of course, natural health advocates the world over

will disagree with my skepticism about diet and brain tumours. Readers should seriously consider the evidence and consult with medically trained practitioners before pursuing any diet cure or treatment. Those particularly interested in the philosophical and ethical issues brought up by this area may be interested in my book *This Book Won't Cure Your Cancer*, which aims to encourage deep thinking about cancer and our attitude to the disease.[26]

Does that mean you should go out and enjoy a high fat, high alcohol, high sugar diet? No, of course not. Though lifestyle and diet have never been pinpointed as a cause or catalyst for brain tumours, they very clearly play a role in the development of other types of cancer, usually indirectly. Smoking is well known as a direct cause of a number of cancers.

One possible exception to my diet skepticism is the Ketogenic diet, which comes in various forms. In many, it is a high fat, low carbohydrate, high protein diet that some claim can reduce the occurrence of epileptic seizures. After fasting, patients cease eating certain starchy vegetables, other starches like bread, pasta and grains, and replace them with butter, cream and nuts. The diet has been shown to make a difference in some children's seizure patterns, as long as it is taken with anti-seizure drugs. But it comes with some serious side effects, such as stunted growth and brittle bones.

The jury is very much out when it comes to adult patients. There's no known effect on brain tumours themselves, either in adults or children. The National Institute for Health and Care Excellence (NICE) in the UK does not recommend the diet for adults. ABTA has a wide ranging webinar about the Ketogenic diet.[27]

Two to 20 years is a pretty broad estimation of when your brain tumour will transform from low grade to malignant, and Duncan Weaver was under no illusion that he might just be on the wrong side of the curve.

It was nearly three years after diagnosis with a low grade brain tumour that his symptoms began to deteriorate so quickly that his doctors became concerned. Within a month and a half, Duncan had gone from being able to do almost everything, to just about being able to walk from the house to the car.

His consultant diagnosed oedema, liquid swelling on the brain that had formed a cyst. It was increasing pressure on his brain, causing seizures and movement problems. Duncan had a three hour operation to release the swelling, and the surgeon implanted a Rickham reservoir – a kind of pool on the skull surface into which excess fluid can drain. That reservoir is then tapped occasionally to remove any build up.

The operation went well, but within weeks Duncan was suffering further seizures. He ended up in accident and emergency, fitting every 20 minutes. The reservoir, which was found to be leaking, had become infected and Duncan had life threatening meningitis. He had to remain in hospital for five weeks, only able to spend a few hours outside during the whole time to celebrate his daughter's birthday.

Throughout this period, doctors had prescribed a powerful steroid to keep swelling and nausea at bay. That led to Duncan developing the so-called 'moon face', where his face blew up. It took many more weeks to wean Duncan off the dexamethasone and for his face to return to normal.

Duncan, Loes and their daughter Tess were then able to enjoy much of a year living in relative normality. Duncan wasn't able to find stable work that could accommodate his needs, but that at least meant he could spend more time with his daughter. He also qualified for various benefits in the Dutch welfare system, which took some of the financial pressure off.

The autumn of 2014, then, was life as normal. He was having physiotherapy sessions, taking time to sleep, then spending the rest of his time with his family. In fact, it was the first incident free period between scans that Duncan had enjoyed since he was first diagnosed. So when they walked into the consultant's room for Duncan's latest routine MRI results, it felt almost like an inconvenient visit.

That's when the neurosurgeon delivered the devastating news. The tumour had started to grow again. And not just by a little. Its speed of growth, said the medic, meant there was little doubt they were now dealing with a high grade tumour. A glioblastoma.

"What does that mean?" Loes had asked through tears.

"For a recurrent astrocytoma?" the doctor had asked himself, aloud. "About one to four years' survival." Chemotherapy would be needed as soon as possible.

The couple felt like they had been hit by a train. The realisation that Duncan would not grow old with this tumour. That the couple would not spend the rest of their lives together. That he would not see their beautiful little girl grow up.

They left the consultant's office in shock. All Duncan and Loes could do was to look at each other and hold each other tight.

Family and friends

"RANT TIME... AFTER my very recent surgery and anaplastic astrocytoma Grade III diagnosis, everyone seems to want a piece of me. 'When can I see you?' Constant text messages. Being asked 101 questions. Constantly being told to be positive because I'm young, fit and healthy. I'm not healthy!!! I have an aggressive unpredictable form of cancer. I have been given an average of five years' life expectancy by my oncologist!! I'm not seen as Sarah anymore, I'm seen as a disease. I am so bloody angry with life and the world."
Sarah Louisa, Facebook post[28]

Thus went a Brain Tumour Charity Facebook post, whose author permitted me to share her words here. She posted them online just two weeks after being diagnosed. Her words and frustration immediately resonated with me, and other posters on the Facebook support page, and will with many other brain tumour patients.

When you are newly diagnosed, all friends and relatives want to do is ask questions and reassure you; all you want to do is crawl under a stone and hide. You feel overwhelmed with information, meanwhile they crave it. Or worse, they think they know better than you about your condition. The result is a mishmash of well meaning but ultimately frustrating back and forth, while you are trying to come to terms with what has happened to you.

As one person posted in response to Sarah Louisa: "Agreed, friends and family do not know how to react. They are trying to show you that they care but [are] not sure what to say or do."

How to solve this dilemma?

A few approaches might work for you or your family, in the short term. First is to write down everything you know about your diagnosis, what might happen now, what is expected in the longer term, and what your own approach to your health and diagnosis is going to be – if you know it. You might also write whether you'd welcome people getting in touch, or whether to ask them to give you some space to gather more information and get initial actions underway.

This is exactly what I did, within days of diagnosis. I circulated it by email, specifically asking people not to get in touch by phone and saying that I'd update them when we knew more. It may have come across as cold and unfriendly, but I excused myself by saying we needed space to process what was going on. It was well received, with only a few breaking the rules and sending me unsolicited nonsense about miracle cures and amazing expert surgeons who would do things no other medic would attempt.

Another approach might be to ask a close friend or family member to become a liaison, some might say a human shield, to provide information about your diagnosis to those who want it. It may well be your partner, but they will be undergoing their own grief and stress, so perhaps you could agree an alternative together. Friends, colleagues and distant relatives could be asked to go through this appointed liaison to pass on their good wishes and questions, while you can flow information through them.

Ultimately, you may decide to keep people informed personally, as your diagnosis shakes down, or via Facebook or email updates. I write a blog, and I know family and friends follow this closely. It saves them the emotional and physical effort of having to continually get in touch, and perhaps risk getting all the latest information upside down or contacting me at a bad time. Or you may decide your mouth is not as big as mine, and prefer to keep all information about your diagnosis, progress and prognosis to yourself.

But the Facebook poster's lament that "I'm not seen as Sarah anymore" is also very relevant. It's a very hard balance to strike for friends and family who I'm not in regular touch with. Obviously, they don't want my cancer's progress to be the first thing they ask about. But they want and need to know. I've become used to the question 'and how are you *getting on?*' (often with a tilt of their head to one side) meaning more than the usual 'hello'. That's fine. I usually quickly sum up the current position, then ask a question about their life, signifying that I'm ready for the conversation to move on.

For people I know less well, especially those who've

heard about my condition on the grapevine, I do fear that, like Sarah Louisa, that I'm seen more as a brain tumour with a body. The answer is perhaps to decide for yourself how open you wish to be about your condition, and whether you wish to share every twist and turn. Or whether you wish to keep the detail to yourself, and try to close down any probing with an 'I'm fine, just getting on with it', which will usually do the trick.

The cheeky answer is to describe another significant aspect of your life – say your kids, sports, or house renovations – as if you've missed the obvious point of their question. That'll soon close down over interested parties you don't want to share your every life turn with. Or you could ask your appointed human shield to spring into action.

As one final Facebook message to Sarah commented: "I am lucky to have so many close friends and family who are asking after me, but find it too tiring and repetitive to answer all messages, even those from very close friends. So I keep people updated on the brain tumour front by keeping a blog, freeing up text/calls/visits for other 'normal' chat. I've said to friends that even if I don't reply, please don't stop sending me messages with news from their end. Good friends will be led by you."

> "I think friends have taken the cue from how we have been reacting over the last ten years. Some have wanted to know all the gory details, while others have been concerned for us and have been there for us when needed."
> Richard Stevens

"My family and friends couldn't have been more supportive and encouraging. I am quite clued in to brain tumour research, clinical studies, and alternative options and both my family and close friends encourage this. I was worried that my brain cancer would define me, but even in my wider circle of acquaintances and colleagues, I was never 'Calum, the guy with the brain tumour' as I had feared."
Calum Wright

James Campling was both frustrated and immensely moved by the way his friends reacted to his glioblastoma.

With a military background, it was no surprise that his RAF colleagues immediately rallied around with support as he went through surgery, then chemotherapy and radiotherapy. Desperate to 'do something' his colleagues began a series of fundraising events for brain tumour research, and it was one of the best reactions he could have hoped for.

But life goes on, and that's hard to take. James's colleagues slowly drifted back to work, back to their own lives. Where once he had shared a social life with his work colleagues, he found himself spending more and more time alone.

Sure, his friends would say 'call anytime', but that's easier said than done. After all, you pick up the phone, call the number, and then what? Try to tell your deepest darkest feelings to someone who's half asleep on the other end of the line?

And anyway, James's loneliest and most frightening times were not in the middle of the night. It was the middle of the day when everyone else was at work that he felt his life ebbing away in front of box sets of old TV dramas.

You should get out more, people would say. Come to this event or that. But motivation is hard when you're waiting for your latest results, and your body feels as if it just stepped out of a boxing ring.

And anyway, James was always conscious that his friends might be uncomfortable: not wanting to talk about their own lives, fearing that their own problems and highlights were nothing compared with the turn his life had taken. His relationship with his friends had changed fundamentally.

Duncan's chemotherapy went well, but he no longer had enough energy to do any work. Meanwhile, his wife Loes was feeling helpless: knowing that chemotherapy could only extend Duncan's life, not prevent his death.

Ever proactive, she decided to join a fundraising event for a Dutch brain tumour charity. Friends and family quickly piled in, and between them 10 people participated in the 25km walk, 25km run, 44km mountain bike, and 125km road cycle.

Not to be outdone, Duncan's friends in the UK took on the Wolf run, an event in our mutual home town of Wolverhampton in aid of The Brain Tumour Charity. The fundraising effort snowballed, and five friends also headed to Amsterdam for the city's marathon. Over eight months, Duncan's friends and family members organised and took part in golf days, tea parties, teddy bear picnics and swimming events.

It was a classic demonstration of how friends and family can deal with the undealable. Knowing they cannot do anything physically to aid our medical condition, friends and family's next instinct is to raise money for charities that are researching treatment and cures.

And the best thing was, Duncan was able to help out with the admin and media side of their fundraising efforts. That gave his life some meaning when he could otherwise have become lost in the drudgery and illness of chemotherapy. It really lifted his spirits to be able to be busy with something so meaningful each day, and by the end of their efforts some £19,000 had been raised for research into brain tumours.

Friends

> "Days before he went into surgery I held my brave beautiful son as he cried in my arms full of fear, but so full of courage. He aced the surgery, but the pathology a couple of weeks later told a different story. The surgeon had found some Grade III cells, and asked if we understood the seriousness of what he was saying. His dad broke down sobbing and had to be removed from the room. Though I was screaming inside, I had to hold it together for George. I did that every day for the next three or more years."
>
> Jane Cooke, mother of George

In my book *Brain Tumours: Living Low Grade*, I outlined different types of reactions from friends to my brain tumour. The rule of thumb categories I came up with resonated so well with the book's readers that they could pretty much slot each of their friends into the boxes I'd created.

Since many of those readers were astrocytoma and glioblastoma patients, I feel able to reproduce those categories here. I hope you feel they do fit and are helpful.

Learning someone you love or know well has a brain tumour or incurable disease does change your relationship with them. It's a cliché to say that terrible news reveals who your friends really are. I think it's a little more nuanced than that. Some friends say: 'Anything I can do?' And they mean it from the bottom of their heart. Others say it because it's the right thing to do, then they get on with their lives.

But I'm hesitant to judge anyone's reaction. The responses will be as diverse as your friends, some expected while others take you by surprise. Some acquaintances will come out of the blue and become solid support, while some great friends will run for the hills. That's cool. People have busy lives, their own priorities, and some people are just better at confronting difficult issues than others.

Yet, I've recognised some patterns that have chimed with other people who have long term illnesses. I must emphasise that I classify them here not in particular judgement, but simply through convenience. Some may cross these categories or end up a combination of some of them, some of the time.

Ignorers

These are the everyday friends and people who you don't necessarily know well, who hear your news for the first time and perhaps send a card telling you to let them know if there's anything they can do. Then you don't hear from them again.

Happy surprisers

These are the friends you wouldn't necessarily have called best buddies, but who then knock you over with their sympathetic, practical and emotional support. Perhaps they've been affected by cancer themselves or just naturally respond well. They come out of the blue with their generosity and understanding and you become very fond of them. It's like discovering new friends all over again.

Rocks

Usually already good friends, these are the guys who simply get it. They're there for you, frequently on the phone, checking in with you but knowing when to give you space too. They understand that it's not just you, but your family and your other friends too who are affected. These are the guys you can call up in the middle of the night. When they turn up to your house to see you, they bring a cake or a pizza and don't expect to be treated like guests. Not because they think you're incapable, but because they know spending time with you is the priority, not cooking and washing up.

These are the guys who come to your bedside when you're about to go into surgery, and who stay with your partner while you're under the knife. They're still there when you come round again. They're the ones who visit you in hospital and pass out news to others so you're not bombarded with phone calls.

Sad surprisers

There will be some friends who you truly believed were some of your closest buddies, but who either can't deal with your diagnosis or appear to be unmoved. They don't call, they don't ask how you are. You don't get the feeling they're there for you and some don't even mention your diagnosis. Some of these guys just don't want to confront an uncomfortable truth or think I don't want to discuss it, so I'm not too hard on them.

Doers

These are the amazing friends – some of whom you will barely know and even their friends who you don't know at all – who do something practical to support one of the brain tumour or cancer charities. They organise a cake sale at work, run a race, cycle long miles or do a sponsored walk, because they want to do something.

Long lost buddies

Some of these are welcome, some not so much. Some will have their own stories to share, others will see an opportunity to rekindle an old friendship. But with others, there may be an unhelpful pressure to meet up, perhaps travel halfway across the country to spend the weekend. It is all meant in good faith, but the sudden onrush of old friends can bring with it a certain burden.

Gossipers

There was one woman in my broader circle of association. She'd never spoken to me in the two years I knew her and I'd not spoken to her. For one reason or another she heard about my diagnosis and suddenly started getting very chatty. Not about brain tumours, but loads of other stuff. She treated me as if we'd been best buddies for years. I'm afraid I couldn't help feeling like I was simply the latest voyeuristic news story.

Brain tumour patients and their families will be inundated with requests of 'how can we help?' by friends and others when they are first diagnosed, and it's a good idea to take advantage of these offers when asked. But perhaps not always immediately.

When I was diagnosed, there wasn't much we initially needed, but we did know there would be times in the future when we would need childcare, a good meal, a short break, or just a coffee and a chat. We made it clear that we were very grateful for all offers, and that when we needed something we would call on them. Don't be afraid to cash in these promises. When you most need them, you'll be glad you held them in reserve. Friends will be delighted to be asked, as all of them really do mean it when they say they want to help.

Partners and family

Some friends come and go, but it is those closest to you – family, partners, spouses – who will have to try to see you through thick and thin as your brain tumour progresses. This is no easy task. The Brain Tumour Charity reports that nine out of ten brain tumour patients become more reliant on others.[29] Two out of three have seen their tumour impact on their relationships with others. This could be because of personality change, or the change in relationship from one of equal partners to carer/cared for.

Simple things patients used to do by themselves – go to the toilet or take a shower – can require assistance, usually from a life partner. This puts emotional strain on the relationship, and can also begin to wear away any remaining sense of intimacy between couples, replacing it with mere physical functionality. One female respondent in the charity's *Losing Myself* report described feeling "inadequate, worthless, a burden, unloved and unlovable".

Apart from the emotional and immediate burden of a brain tumour diagnosis upon a loved one, there are also wider practical implications to consider. One particular hardship, for example, is the continual visits to doctors and hospitals which you may not be able to, or wish to, attend by yourself. Another is their need to assist or fill in for you with children, cooking and social engagements, when you're struck by extreme fatigue. Both of these may demand a loved one taking time off work or away from other aspects of life, spending long hours in waiting rooms, shuffling childcare, hobbies and other commitments, to be with a patient.

While it is all done generously and with love, it shouldn't be underestimated that this caring responsibility puts great pressure on a loved one. Most difficult, perhaps, is the feeling that they can't complain – after all, you're the one with the brain tumour. They just have to drive the car or sit next to you while you wait. It is important that those supporting people with brain tumours do not feel this way. Indeed, the better they are supported themselves, the better they will be able to assist the patient.

The first step is for carers to allow themselves to feel annoyed and guilty and frustrated, because these feelings are very real and legitimate. The next is to look at how to manage the new responsibilities imposed upon them. Perhaps family members could consider drawing up a rota of hospital visits, to ensure the burden of work and lifts doesn't fall upon the same person all of the time. Childcare can be shared, meals cooked and dropped round. In some countries and states, financial benefits are available to those who find themselves in a caring position.

> "Sometimes it seems like Liz has had to act more like a parent than a partner. I forget things very easily these days. As my maths is rubbish it is much easier for her to make quick decisions about simple money issues. She does make a lot of decisions generally off her own bat, not all of which I would have agreed to! For more important decisions then we make those together; it is just that these take longer than they used to as I need time to figure things out. We have not talked much about the inevitable. It will end up with her becoming more and more the boss. As we really do not know how things will progress we will need to make more specific plans as the time comes. I do not want to become a burden."
> Richard Stevens

> "Every night when I went to bed, I wondered if Sue would still be there in the morning. I found it impossible to make any preparations, suffering from anticipatory grief. I was sick with terror. I couldn't sleep properly and I lost 8kg. "
> Joanna Waters, sister of Sue Rossides

Separation

The simple truth is that some intimate relationships cannot stand the strain, and separation can become inevitable. Brain tumour patients I have spoken to, and their loved ones, have not expressed that they have fallen out of love with their partner, but that the love has had to change and move on. In many cases, their sexual and intimate life has been profoundly affected. Sometimes the resultant split is amicable, sometimes the patient – or their partner – feels abandoned in their time of most need.

There are no easy answers to these quandaries, and they can sometimes be made even more complex by the presence of young or teenage children. Charities can provide some support, but it will be for each couple to decide what intervention they wish to pursue: from friends and their wider family, to accessing counselling or legal help.

If there is any word of comfort to be shared, it is that before the brain tumour those relationships were real and meaningful, and will always carry with them good memories. It is hard not to let current or future hurt overwrite history, so taking good note of the great times, with photographs and videos as keepsakes, will help both patient and loved ones to remember life before the illness began to intervene.

Some couples and relationships, of course, become stronger as a result of being challenged by illness. Indeed, some blossom as partners fall into roles that feel natural to them: carer, cared for, loving support, cook, gatekeeper. Ultimately, relationships are as wide and diverse as the brains in which tumours grow. But for those who find they cannot cope, support is available.

Duncan Weaver and his wife Loes were committed to taking on his brain tumour together. They had only been married for three months when he was diagnosed, and now they were nearly four years on with toddler Tess bouncing around in the mix.

But that didn't mean it was easy for the couple. As well as Duncan's illness, and his difficulty finding work, Loes had her own problems. The company she worked with announced it would close its offices in the Netherlands, leaving her looking for work. As she was filling out application forms and polishing up her CV, she was at the same time seeing Duncan deteriorate and wondering if she'd be able to take on any job she was offered anyway.

Duncan, once great with words, no longer had the language skills to help her. He simply couldn't get his head around what he was trying to say. He'd lose his train of thought easily, then when he gained it again, Loes might have moved on. That made him angry because he thought she'd stopped listening to him.

In fact, anger was something Duncan was finding increasingly difficult to manage. Whether down to the medication, the brain tumour, the stress or a combination of these things, he developed a really bad temper. Friends never saw it, but with Loes and Tess it could be over even the smallest, most insignificant thing. She sometimes resented his friends only seeing the good side of him, but then felt guilty about that resentment. In her own way, Loes' life was collapsing too.

Their physical intimacy had all but gone away, complicated by medication and fatigue. But much more, Loes realised she badly missed her best friend. The person with whom she could talk about anything, the one who understood her best, the one with whom a glance or a single word was enough, the one with whom she had had so much fun. She missed her husband.

But on the flip side, the couple felt stronger than ever about each other. A bond had developed that, wherever they were going, they were going there together. That single glance or single word was still there. They were determined to try to make as much of their time together as they could.

Telling young children

Anaplastic astrocytoma in particular, as well as the occasional *de novo* glioblastoma, does affect people in their 30s and 40s. That means some patients may well find they have their own young children living at home who will perhaps have to cope with their illness, even death. For older patients, they may have grandchildren who will have to deal with the diagnosis.

How can you begin to think about telling children that you have a brain tumour, that you might die? Or should you not tell them at all?

When I was diagnosed, and at that time it was assumed my life expectancy would be quite short, my wife and I decided quite quickly that we would not hide anything from our (then) two children. They were just two and four at the time, and wouldn't have managed a 'sit down, we have something to tell you' conversation. But we decided to drop the idea of brain tumours into general conversation, that Daddy had one, that I was sick and tired a lot of time, that I had to go to hospital a lot, and that I had seizures a lot of the time.

They absorbed knowledge by osmosis as we simply went about our business of dealing with the disease.

They have both grown up knowing nothing else except that Daddy is seriously ill, and while I think that will stay with them for the rest of their lives, the alternative – that they suddenly discover something so devastating and that we've been hiding it from them for years – is unthinkable. Now seven and nine, they're much more able to comprehend the idea that my brain tumour might mean I'm not around forever, though I don't think they have a strong idea of death and what it really means. Occasionally we drop into deeper conversations about what will happen, and whether I will die from my brain tumour, and we all generally conclude that none of us can really know what's going to happen into the future.

Since diagnosis, we have had another baby, and we feel the approach we've taken is so right for us as a family that it will be the same with our new toddler as she grows up.

That is not to say our way is the best. Some parents want to hide their diagnosis from their children entirely, fearing perhaps they will no longer be seen as 'Mum' or 'Dad', but as an incapable parent or something not quite right or broken. It is for every parent to decide for themselves. Some patients have very good reasons to keep their diagnosis quiet.

But if you do attempt to talk to your children about cancer, or about your brain tumour in particular, at what age is most appropriate, and how should you go about it? Will you even have a choice, if you are sporting new scars on your head, have lost hair, or have to take a long spell in hospital?

Once again, charities and support groups will be the most helpful here. The Brain Tumour Charity in the UK has developed a series of upbeat animated films, one of the best of which is called *Mummy has a brain tumour*, which takes a no-nonsense approach to Mummy's diagnosis, behaviour changes, the treatment she undergoes, and finishes with ultimate uncertainty about what might happen next.[30] It is the most useful thing I have shown my children about my condition. I particularly like it because it does not attempt to tell children that Mummy will be okay in the end, but reflects the ongoing uncertainty that necessarily comes with the disease.

Another large British cancer charity, Macmillan Cancer Support, publishes an extensive brochure on telling children and teenagers about cancer.

"Being honest and including them in what's happening is usually the best approach," the booklet says. "When the time comes, many parents find the conversation more natural and less traumatic than they expected."[31]

Macmillan advises parents to consider the age of their children, and to speak to each one on terms that they will understand and not find scary. A five year old boy might envisage some intergalactic war taking place in your head, while a teenager is likely to be much more engaged in the distress that it causes you and the rest of the family. Be prepared for children to take time to understand, to want to be on their own, to be seemingly cold or unfeeling, or to break down.

Ultimately, you will know your children best and will take the best approach, appropriate to your relationship with them. Things to consider might be: whether to take them to your doctor and hospital appointments; whether to share pictures of your MRI scans; whether to show them any picc line you have (a thin plastic tube left under your skin to deliver chemotherapy drugs into your body) or any sites where injections have taken place; whether to show them any medication you're taking at home (with all the necessary precautions); and whether to teach them, or remind them of, emergency procedures for calling an ambulance or the doctor.

The charity says children given news such as this are likely to temporarily revert to being more clingy or to doing things you thought they had outgrown, and that they might think they have done something wrong to cause the problem. This is particularly so if you have become stressed, edgy or more easily lose your temper than you did before diagnosis. It's important to reassure them that your brain tumour is not their fault, not to use your illness as an excuse for poor parenting, and to try to keep regular family routines to bring normality back when it feels right.

In extreme circumstances, child psychologists and family counselling services may help you to tackle even the most difficult issues with your children. Don't be afraid to call upon help if you need it. Allow children to express their feelings, using painting, craft, writing, clay modelling, or whatever other equipment they have. You'll be amazed what they come up with. I still keep some of my kids' earliest brain tumour related drawings, both because they're very special but also because they show even their earliest understanding of my illness and what it does to me.

If it becomes clear that your brain tumour is beginning to become a threat to your life, there are perhaps more intimate things you may consider doing with or for your children. You might consider, for example, putting a memory box together with them: a shoe box or similar, decorated together, full of ticket stubs, photographs, jewellery, receipts, poems and books you've shared together.

Another approach, which may be cathartic for both you and your children, may be to begin taking video of you together, sharing simple things like a meal, a day out, or even the journey to school. You may wish to make personal videos for each child, talking about what you like most about them, what you think they may become in the future (though not instructing them what they must become!), and telling them that you loved and will always love them.

Ultimately, says Macmillan Cancer Support, "cancer may bring some positive things to your family life. Being open and honest with your children can make you feel closer. You can feel proud of how your children have learned to cope when life doesn't go to plan. And don't be afraid to say how proud you are of them."

Experts also agree that when a patient dies, it is unwise to tell children that they have 'gone to sleep'. This may put the child in fear of falling asleep themselves, as well as in expectation that their loved one will one day wake up. They advise using straightforward terms like 'death', or 'passed away', though those from a spiritual background may have their own messages to pass on to children.

Telling parents

In contrast, or in addition, you may find that as a newly diagnosed glioblastoma or anaplastic astrocytoma patient, that you have parents to tell about your situation. I was 35 when I had to call my parents from outside the hospital, next to a loud and busy main road, to tell them first about the seizures I had been having – I'd kept those a secret – and then that I had a brain tumour.

Luckily for me, my parents were relatively young and recently retired, rather than elderly. I wasn't in a caring role, so telling them was emotional but it did not have implications for any support I was providing for them. I was lucky enough to be able to talk to them adult to adult, just as I would with friends who had a deep love and kinship with me. I know my diagnosis affected them both deeply, but the implications were not wider than our emotional relationship.

For many brain tumour patients, however, things will be far more complex. Some older patients, for example, may have parents who have their own needs due to frailty, dementia, cancer or any other condition that can be more prevalent in older people. This is particularly true in primary glioblastoma patients, for whom the diagnosis age tends to be over 55.

How can you tell someone for whom *you* provide care and support, that you are going to need care and medical interventions yourself? How can you communicate your diagnosis to an older relative who is perhaps themselves experiencing memory, cognitive or physical disabilities?

These are very complex questions, the answer for which will depend on the family, its physical and emotional makeup, and the roles each of you currently play. It is certain that things will have to change if you undergo treatment for your brain tumour, so it will be very difficult to keep the news from an older loved one. You are advised to ask for advice not only from your own medical team, but also from any medical or social services team responsible for your parents.

This is again perhaps where close friends and family, as well as brain tumour support groups, can be of particular use. If you have brothers and sisters, for example, is there a strategy that you can put together for telling and supporting your parents, and redistributing any caring responsibilities you have previously taken on?

The cancer and brain tumour charities may be able to help you plan ahead financially, to see if you can get extra help for yourself and for your parents, given your drastically changed circumstances. If nothing else, other members will have been through the same experiences and will have ideas, strategies and support to share.

One piece of advice is to decide on how much you wish to share with your parents. You may wish to protect them from all the details, or you may wish to open up completely, but it is your decision to make. Many cancer patients wait for a little while, until they have begun to digest the news themselves, before telling their parents. Sometimes they may wait for any physical indications, such as loss of hair or having to undergo treatment, to break the news.

It is probably wise to avoid attempting to second guess what a parent's response will be. Like you, it is very likely they would want to know. They will want to be given the chance to digest the information, question, understand, then try to offer mutual support as you deal with the diagnosis together into the future. But at the same time, it is important that you understand how these particular brain tumours work before attempting to embark on an explanation to potentially vulnerable people such as elderly parents, who may become scared and anxious more easily.

The brain tumour community

As someone experiencing a brain tumour, as a patient or loved one, you will have your own sources of family and friendship support, as well as support recommended to you by your clinical and hospice advisors.

It is also worth noting the huge amount of support that is available through what has become known as the 'brain tumour community'. This is the informal conglomeration of charities, support groups, Facebook and talkboard groups, buddying projects and other ways of sharing for those who have been affected by the disease. These groups are far from just for patients.

Before I was diagnosed, I think I'd probably only read about brain tumours in sensationalist news stories, usually when a celebrity was affected. After diagnosis, an underworld of hundreds, perhaps thousands of people appeared. Each of them had stories to tell, advice to impart, experiences to share. A newcomer was welcomed with open and loving arms, but only as far as they wanted to venture. There was no pressure to join, or turn up, or to contribute.

The beauty of this broad community is that we can access the support we want when we need it, and how we need it. In some cases, there are helplines with a real human voice at the other end, usually an expert in brain tumours who may have been through some of the experiences we have. Or they will know others who have. In other cases, perhaps you will have a question about your diagnosis that you can't get your doctor to answer. A Facebook post will create a wealth of opinions and evidence based answers, as well as some funny and warm hearted responses, that will help. Sure, there's debate and disagreement, just as you would find in any community, but it's done with a mutual understanding of what we all have to go through.

Lian stumbled across a brain tumour site for carers on Facebook that, she says, was a godsend in her darkest days. All of a sudden she realised she wasn't alone. Others had relatives with the same. Children had brain tumours. The disease didn't discriminate.

From that moment, she stopped feeling sorry for herself and her family. Her attitude changed. She still felt alone, but didn't obsess as much.

On your lowest days, just reading Facebook or talkboard responses to other people's questions will remind you that you are not alone. You can usually find answers to your query and encounter some surprises without even asking a question.

That's because others have been through what you are going through. They know things that you don't and are willing to share. They are advocates for better treatment, better diagnosis and better understanding of brain tumours. In a medicalised world, the brain tumour community illustrates that the disease affects human beings with empathetic hearts who are willing to share and support each other with what they know. I hope this book too contributes to that approach.

Prognosis

LIAN'S MOTHER'S TUMOUR began growing back almost immediately after her initial surgery, but she survived for a further three years. During that time, Gillian was offered nurses but Lian was determined: her mother had had three children, and she had always looked after them. Now they would do what they could for her.

But it did become tiring. At the beginning, Gillian's partner was good in the day but wanted nights off to sleep; otherwise he would get short with her mum. As things got really tough, he started to disengage, spending more time in the pub than at home. Perhaps it was his way of coping, Lian didn't know. She tried to stay positive, but the pressure pot sometimes boiled over.

Lian lived a couple of doors down from her mum, so it was easier for her to go and see her than her sister, who had a house full of children. Her brother couldn't do the personal care Gillian needed, so much of it fell on the elder sister. At times she would sleep on her mum's sofa, so she could help when Gillian woke in the night needing to use the toilet.

She knew her siblings were doing what they could, but she couldn't help feeling resentment when she thought someone wasn't pulling their weight.

The nurses began suggesting hospice visits, but Lian was totally against it. It felt like giving up. But when she properly came to understand what her mother was being offered – to have her hair done, a hand massage, to spend time with others in similar circumstances – she agreed with her siblings that it would be a lovely and positive rather than negative thing.

As soon as Lian and her family knew they were going to lose Gillian, they vowed to create some special memories for her, and for themselves. Gillian's birthday came along not long after her diagnosis, so it was a perfect opportunity to start the tradition. The family didn't have too much cash, but what they lacked in money they made up for in effort. They took over the corner of an Indian restaurant, put up balloons, brought their own sparkling wine, invited guests to prepare for the surprise event. Lian had even asked some buskers from outside the shopping centre whether they'd play.

It was such a simple evening, but when Gillian walked through the door and everyone cheered and the live band struck up, the smile on her face was worth a million spent on any glittering occasion. Even the band joined the party, sitting down with the guests.

That night the whole family swore they would make each of their mother's remaining birthdays better than the last. However much money you have, memories are the best thing you can own.

It is natural for patients, their family and loved ones, to ask their doctors: 'how long have I got?' Their response, if they offer one at all, is likely to be no more than an estimation. They can only speak from personal experience, the scientific papers they have read, and base their opinion on your own health, age, tumour type, its size, position, success of treatment and any number of other factors.

Prognosis cannot be projected forward. Patients, doctors and researchers can only look back to what has happened to patients with your condition over time *in the past*. In some cases, a picture of probable life expectancies can be built. In others, we are all grasping in the dark. Some people live for much longer than initially projected, and others less. Nothing is set in stone.

However, this chapter does contain hard (and hard to stomach) statistics on the prognosis of patients with anaplastic astrocytoma and glioblastoma. You may wish to stop for a moment and consider whether you want to continue reading.

Some patients do not want to know what their chances are, and ask their loved ones to keep that information from them. Sometimes it works the other way: with patients desperate to share and make the most of the time they may have left, but with loved ones refusing to hear or acknowledge the possibility that the tumour cannot be cured.

The people I worked with on this book, patients and family, were generous enough to share their own experiences. This area appeared to be the most frustrating and painful one to speak about, so it should come as no surprise if you feel nervous to read on.

There are a few things to note before we begin to understand prognosis properly, and a few provisos that you must read after the statistics to properly understand them.

First to note is that, when you are looking at scientific papers about survival, you will need to know the difference between progression free survival (PFS) and overall survival (OS). PFS indicates that a patient's life has continued, essentially unchanged, after an initial intervention such as treatment, or from diagnosis. That is not the same as OS, which is the sum total of the patient's life from diagnosis – whatever the quality of that life may be. A patient may enjoy a year of PFS before another six months of further treatment, disability, poor quality of life and eventual death. The totality of this is their OS.

Second to note is that you should take very specific care to read up on and understand any prognosis you are given, or that you read in scientific papers, on the internet, in books such as this, or in information from charities. Sometimes it might feel like you need a statistics degree to understand what you are being told.

For example, cancer prognosis is often expressed as 'median five year survival'. Do you know what this means? A classic mistake would be to understand it as the patient having a 50 percent chance of surviving for five years. But that is not what 'median' means. Remember, statistics are mainly based on looking back. A 'median five year survival' means: of the group studied, 50 percent were still alive after five years, and 50 percent had died.

Another mistake would be to project this five year survival as a straight and constant line: that the longer time goes on, the more patients will die in a pretty regular and predictable pattern. This isn't necessarily the case. Those patients who have survived for five years may well be the ones who are likely to survive for far longer. Perhaps the patients before the median were frail and already quite ill, while those who survived the median tended to be younger, fitter and with more options for their treatment.

In short, it is important to look at the studies that have produced the statistics, not just the statistics themselves, to get an accurate picture of your own case. If in doubt, ask your doctors.

Also, some studies are based on very small numbers of patients, so you should be wary of drawing too many implications from them. Others include only young patients. Or only older patients. Or are assessments of tumours that are different from yours. Previously they might have been relevant to your tumour, but the progress of genetic analysis of tumours – as you will learn about later – has now made those earlier studies irrelevant to the particular type of tumour you have.

Third to note is that new studies are being carried out all the time. Not only brand new clinical trials and analyses, but old data is being revisited with new techniques and definitions, to produce new data about prognosis. What I write here may not be relevant or correct by the time you read it. Statistics used by organisations tend to lag behind realtime research. In all cases, you should follow up on the original sources to see if anything has changed since I gathered the information together.

It's also worth noting that sources don't always agree. That is the nature of scientific research and study. Some centres consider different factors as important; they make judgements based on different studies, statistics and assumptions.

It is in our nature to look for the best case scenario, but it's not helpful when we get three different prognosis predictions, from three different organisations, for the same condition. Who to believe? The answer is that you can only ever get a very broad impression of prognosis from statistics. The real answer is likely to lie in what your doctors and your own body are telling you, and how you respond to what they advise.

> "I'm undoubtedly privileged to have even lived
> my life but I'm still young, naïve and wanting
> 101 different things. The approximation is I've
> now a 27% chance to go further than five
> more years. Visualising myself removed from
> those statistics is becoming a much harder task
> with the startling progression some scans
> present, from one to the next."
> Jack Webb

Prognosis for these brain tumours

Because these tumours are apt to grow into surrounding tissue, anaplastic astrocytomas and glioblastomas can be very difficult to treat. Without treatment, these aggressive tumour cells multiply rapidly. In almost all cases, they are fatal.

As a very general rule, the more incapacitated a patient is when they are diagnosed, the less time they are likely to survive. This is measured by something called the Karnofsky Performance Score (KPS), which measures a person's functional capability and ability to move independently, as well as their cognitive ability. Essentially, KPS indicates a person's ability to care for themselves.

A low score means a patient has a low ability to care for themselves, as well as poor motor and cognitive skills. Someone with a low KPS, generally regarded as lower than 60 on a scale of 0-100, has poorer prospects. Those with a score higher than 60 have better prospects. Doctors will often use KPS to help make decisions about proposed treatments, and whether they are likely to be useful.

Whatever your situation, it is unlikely you, or a loved one, will die within weeks of diagnosis. From various reliable medical and expert sources, the following predictions and prognoses are recorded for anaplastic astrocytoma and glioblastoma. And in all cases, there are outliers: patients who have continued to live many, many years, despite having apparently the most aggressive tumours. The opposite is also the case.

The following is very broad brush and tends to be drawn from studies of all patients with the following types of tumour. As well as KPS, different genetic factors within these tumours can be predictive of better or worse outcomes than outlined here. It is important to understand how the genetic makeup of tumours works to get a more accurate prediction.

Anaplastic astrocytoma

The American Brain Tumor Association (ABTA) records that the expected median survival rate for adults with this tumour type is two to three years from diagnosis. This is presuming the patient has all the normal treatment: usually surgery, followed by radiotherapy and chemotherapy.[32] This means that half of adult patients will have passed away after two to three years, while half will remain alive.

Taking their information from the National Cancer Information Network (a United States organisation), Cancer Research UK says more than 20 out of 100 people with Grade III astrocytoma survive their disease for five years or more after they are diagnosed.[33]

According to The Brain Tumour Charity in the UK, about one in four people (27 percent) diagnosed with a high grade astrocytoma live for five years or more.[34]

Glioblastoma

Adult patients with this more aggressive tumour have poorer chances, even with the standard treatment of aggressive surgery, radiation and temozolomide chemotherapy, says ABTA.[35] Half of patients will have passed away after nearly 15 months from diagnosis. Only one in ten patients will live for five years.

Cancer Research UK says: around five out of 100 people with Grade IV astrocytoma survive their disease for five years or more after they are diagnosed. The organisation's prognosis for children with these brain tumours is far more favourable, though cases are rare.[36]

According to The Brain Tumour Charity in the UK, the average survival time is 12-18 months. Only two in ten glioblastoma patients survive more than one year, and only three percent of patients survive more than three years.

All of the above reinforces what I have already written: that there is a significant variance in the statistics, and every patient is different. The patterns point in a particular direction, but patterns are not predictions of any particular patient's prognosis. Indeed, any talk of prognosis must come with a long list of caveats, and I must make it clear that this book makes no attempt at all to predict your own, or your loved ones' chances. I aim to honestly report science based information from my own research.

When looking at the statistics above, and any other information you encounter on prognosis, you should always consider the 'ifs' and 'buts'. No prognosis comes without provisos.

Proviso 1 – You are not a number

You'll hear it a hundred times. No brain tumour patient is the same. Your tumour has its own size, type, genetic makeup, position, activity level, malignancy and impact on your brain. Your age and KPS is not the same as another's. This does not mean you are 'bound to buck the trend' as some patients say they are (frustratingly) told. It means prognosis based on past studies can only ever be very broad in indicating your own tumour journey. It cannot define it. Nevertheless, if you have a brain tumour that has been studied in detail, any prognosis will be based on good science.

Proviso 2 – We look for the most hopeful

We have a tendency to look for the best news, and stick to it. It is of course true that we should seek second, third and even fourth opinions on our prognosis, as well as seek out further information about our tumour type. We should avoid, however, finding the best case scenario and then deciding that it must be the truth. If a different doctor gives us a better prognosis, what reason should we have to listen to them rather than the one who has given us only months to live? The internet can be a real chasm in this respect, so patients and loved ones are advised to proceed with caution.

Proviso 3 – Hindsight is wonderful, and frustrating

So often in my encounters with brain tumour patients over the last five years have I read words to the tune of: "Doctors gave him three months, he lasted three years", or contrarily: "They said she had very good survival chances, but she died within a week." Both come with understandable passionate emotions, and often a desperate call for justice, an apology or compensation. Though it is not my place to defend or prosecute doctors, it is worth reiterating that these are very serious, very unpredictable brain tumours. In most cases, doctors just don't know. In the same way as we should take their predictions and prognoses with due care, we should similarly be wary of laying blame at their door should their prognosis be wildly wrong.

Proviso 4 – Testimony doesn't mean truth

It is a personal frustration of mine, but I know it is one shared by other brain tumour patients. People who discover you have a brain tumour often tell you stories of friends, or most often *friends of friends*, who have beaten the odds and are surviving well beyond what was predicted for them. Sometimes, it is claimed, they are completely cured. If they can do it, so can you! Some complementary and alternative medicine websites, books and gurus also seem to have unlimited stories of those who have survived against the odds.

Once again it is worth remembering that each

patient is different, that we tend to want to cling to the best news possible, and that those who have not survived beyond their predicted prognosis don't tend to be highlighted as 'incredible stories'. At the risk of sounding a bore, you should consult your physician with any stories like these, particularly if the survival is purported to be the result of some particular treatment you have not had.

As with most diffuse astrocytomas, Duncan Weaver was given temozolomide as a first chemotherapy line of defence. The treatment went well, with few side effects except the expected fatigue and occasional nausea. Thankfully, it didn't make Duncan's seizures any worse and he was still relatively mobile after adapting to his numb right leg.

But after three four-week cycles of temozolomide, Duncan and Loes headed again for the MRI machine, and then the consultant's office. It was not good news. The chemotherapy had had no effect at all. Doctors won't give treatment that doesn't work. The chemotherapy regime would be stopped.

Over the next year, Duncan underwent an ever changing regime of brain tumour treatment and experienced umpteen side effects and illnesses. He returned for some further 30 sessions of radiotherapy. Waiting for the MRIs following Duncan's second round of radiotherapy was the toughest time of all (doctors only usually allow one round, because it can be so tough on the brain).

The first MRI after the radiotherapy had shown growth in the tumour, but that could have been general scarring caused by the radiotherapy itself. The second MRI, after nine months, was when they would find out whether the treatment had worked. It was a very long nine months.

Duncan took various medication and interventions to deal with the side effects of the treatments he was having. His steroids kept him awake at night, but hardly able to function during the day. He developed oedema in the brain again, creating more serious seizures than ever before.

A couple of times they were so fierce he ended up in the accident and emergency department, with medics trying to bring his fitting body under control with sedatives. Duncan started using a mobility scooter to get around, with walking long distances just becoming too much. Even using the *bakfiets* bike was no longer possible, cutting Duncan off from the school run he'd appreciated so much because it gave him time and a connection with his daughter.

He developed diabetes from the long term use of steroids, so had to take more drugs for that. He lost his appetite completely, eating only a little to accompany his family, but neither enjoying nor wanting it.

Duncan was on 19 different tablets a day. Even the biggest pill boxes couldn't fit his doses. Loes used a craft hobby box instead to make sure he got the right drug, in the right dose, at the right time.

Previously, the couple had been simply unwilling to give up. Believing in positive scenarios had been the only way they could cope with the disease. Constantly fearing the negative would be not much of a life at all.

Eventually, they came to a point where they had to be realistic and prepare themselves for the possibility that no treatment was going to work. Slowly resignation crept in.

What if there is tumour recurrence?

Different types of these tumours are more likely to grow back, and some faster than others. Depending on their genetic makeup, even a particular type of glioblastoma is likely to give a patient much more time before recurrence than another type.

Glioblastomas can and do sit dormant for years for some patients, though those cases would be exceptional. One person interviewed for this book has been living post-treatment for glioblastoma for five years and is going strong.

Anaplastic astrocytomas are far more likely to go dormant for a time after treatment, and medical protocols have patients first on a three month MRI monitoring protocol, dropping to six months and then even to a year.

But what happens when a tumour does reoccur? The answer varies from country to country, and even hospital to hospital, though neurologists and oncologists do meet every year to share, critique and hammer out new research and try to establish standard practice.

The National Comprehensive Cancer Network (NCCN) in the United States offers a good impression of treatment pathways for different tumour types, and what the standard practice tends to be after diagnosis; and then later if there is recurrence. The NCCN publishes a detailed guide for clinicians on the latest research and indicates the different recommended treatment pathways. Thankfully, they also publish an easier to understand patient guide which is well worth a read.[37] The UK has its own brain cancer guidelines, published by its own National Institute for Health and

Care Excellence (NICE).[38]

The various pathways the two organisations suggest indicate treatment and responses dependent on how possible surgery is, how a patient responds to treatment, what chemotherapy they are able to tolerate, as well as their age and KPS score, and then based on whether the tumour recurs or not. You are advised to have a closer look at the guidelines for your own country, relating to your own tumour and its responses to treatment. You may get a good impression of why your doctors are suggesting what they are, and on what basis and protocols they are working.

The options are complex, and little is set in stone. But this shows that doctors are following some kind of guidelines when they make decisions about what treatment or care you should consider. And these guidelines are based on sound scientific evidence, not guesswork.

Can we beat the odds?

> "I had to tell my son when they first diagnosed the tumour. Now I had to tell my son as gently as possible that they would stop treatment.
> With such courage he looked at me and said, 'Oh well'. I looked at the heart monitor and it had gone from 56 to 146. My own heart broke in that second."
> Jane Cooke, mother of George

There must be something a patient can do to improve their life chances, right? This is a difficult question to answer. In a sense, a patient can beat the odds by being the *right kind* of patient. That means, patients with certain factors will tend to live longer and have a higher quality of life than others. For example, younger patients (those under 40), those with good cognition and mobility (high KPS), those who have smaller tumours, those who have the most debulking of their tumours, as well as those whose tumours do not cross between the two sides of the brain and have not spread, tend to do better than patients who do not meet these factors.

Of course, this doesn't really tell you how to *beat* the odds, but simply how the odds apply to you as a particular patient. The odds, or more accurately the statistics, are based on this information. They don't influence it. This is a difficult concept to understand, but it's crucial.

So, can we do anything to *improve* our chances? This is where I must duck out and refer to higher powers – whatever you regard them to be: doctors, religious leaders, nature therapists, oncologists or whoever you are most likely to believe. Some brain tumour patients put their extended survival down to the very precise, very expert work of their medical doctors, who they believe diagnosed them early, gave them exactly the right treatment at the right time, and have done everything right to create the best outcome possible. Others may say exactly the opposite of the very same doctor.

Other brain tumour patients may find their doctor useless, even though they've received the right treatment, but put their prolonged survival down to diet, or exercise, or meditation, or religion. Other brain tumour patients and their families talk of 'fighting' their tumours, not giving up, the power of positive thinking and mindfulness.

But whatever we believe, there is one sad fact that we cannot escape. We are already part of the statistics, we cannot sit outside of them. A diagnosis of a brain tumour may well come with a 12 month prognosis. But that 12 months will be based on statistics that have been generated looking at the life expectancies and eventual outcomes of many patients. That means those who unexpectedly live much longer have *already been accounted for* in predicting life expectancy for others. They're not bucking the odds, they're part of the maths that have gone into creating the odds.

It means that all of those living much longer than expected – whether down to great oncology, great exercise and diet, or eating turmeric – are already factored into the statistics.

None of this is intended to put a downer on anyone's hopes, or to urge you to give up the 'fight' against your brain tumour. We all need hope, goals and achievements to get through the days, weeks, months and years. Sometimes hope is all we have, and if we can make the most of this, celebrating each little victory, then all the better for us and our families as we cope with the disease.

It's hard, but for me: I have to believe that all is never lost. That I'll keep on keeping on. That's why I'm writing this book. That's why I ride my bike. That's why I spend as much time with my kids as I can. That's why I try to live as normally as possible. It's vital for maintaining good mental health. What else am I supposed to do but do the things that make me, *me*?

The importance of genetics

This is an exciting time for brain tumour research and

treatment, after many years of underfunding. At the forefront of this research is a better understanding of the genetic and molecular makeup of these tumours. It is influencing how doctors can predict survival times, and dictating what treatments are advised for different tumours.

In 2016, the World Health Organization (WHO) published a new overview of the definition of different types of brain tumours. The previous version, published some 10 years before, concentrated on how tumours looked under the microscope. To understand the huge step forward between then and now, it's necessary to understand a little of what went on before.

The 2007 WHO Classification of Tumours of the Central Nervous System defined tumours mainly according to their 'histology' – the shape of brain tumour cells, and their behaviour. From close examination, using chemical dyes and other techniques (called 'morphology'), researchers were able to tell patients that they had a certain type of brain tumour: say an anaplastic astrocytoma, or a glioblastoma.[39]

The more abnormal the cell looked and behaved, the higher the grade ascribed to the tumour. This allowed oncologists to define the difference between a low grade astrocytoma, which might sport pretty regular astrocytic cells, and a high grade astrocytoma, the cells of which would look highly abnormal. A glioblastoma's cells would be even more abnormal, and would be proliferating hugely.

Thus a patient was able to be told what type of tumour they had: an astrocytoma Grade II, an astrocytoma Grade III or an anaplastic astrocytoma, or a glioblastoma (or else, some other kind of brain tumour). For some time, this histological grading of brain tumours was more or less as good as it got, and oncologists would make an estimation of the right type of treatment to use for each grade and type.

But slowly, scientists began to understand that brain tumours also have specific genetic structures. That means that brain tumour cells might either contain or lack a particular sequence of genes in their DNA, or that genetic sequences might have been swapped around or cut short.

They noticed that brain tumours with or without a particular 'genetic signature' tended to respond to different treatment more or less positively. It appeared that what mattered wasn't just the grade or type of tumour the patient had, but the genetics in the tumour too.

In short, calling a tumour a glioblastoma was no longer enough. One patient might have a glioblastoma that had a particular genetic dysfunction, and therefore was very responsive to chemotherapy, while another might lack that dysfunction and chemotherapy wouldn't be relevant to them. In fact, it might introduce negative side effects for the patient but bring none of the benefits hoped for.

As the science progressed, scientists, academics and oncologists began to use this newly emerging data to more accurately diagnose tumours than from just looking at the histology. And depending on the histology and the genetic and molecular structure, they would act according to their own latest reading and research to recommend the most effective treatment.

It is too much to say this happened on an *ad hoc* basis, but medics' responses to tumours certainly varied. In 2016, the WHO gathered together all the latest research and data to publish a new classification system for brain tumours. Out went the generalised Grade I, II, III and IV (though the terms are still used) and in came very specific names for tumour types, with their various genetic makeup accounted for. Actually, it has become a complex numbering system like the library Dewey decimal system.

A few examples should suffice. My own brain tumour would previously have been judged – on the old system – as a Grade III oligodendroglioma, onto which my oncologist would have attached the outcome of the genetic testing carried out on the tumour.

In my case, they would have identified from the cell structure that it was an oligodendroglioma (the cells look like fried eggs), and from their behaviour (under the microscope, as well as the tumour's behaviour on MRI) as a Grade III. From genetic testing, they have identified two important molecular patterns. My tumour has a piece of DNA missing from two of its strands. This produces the genetic signature of '1P/19Q deletion'.

Another gene which can go wrong in brain tumours in called IDH1. When it does malfunction, it creates a similarly malfunctioning IDH1 enzyme. This scrambling of the gene and its enzyme produces a genetic signature of the tumour called 'IDH mutation'. It is actually very common to have an oligodendroglioma that is 1P/19Q and IDH mutant, but not all oligodentrogliomas have both of these signatures. In fact, those that do are given one type of chemotherapy, and those that don't may be given another. Those that do have 1P/19Q and IDH mutant genes tend to respond better to treatment than those that don't.

This information has been known for a long time,

but the last two guidelines published by the World Health Organization have also created new numbered labels for specific tumours. An oligodendroglioma Grade III, 1P/19Q deletion, IDH mutant is known as: 9451/3.

In the new system, the previous terms are also used along with the numbers. So to give my tumour it's full title, it is an: *oligodendroglioma, IDH-mutant and 1p/19q-codeleted, 9451/3*.

Another example: glioblastoma brain tumours that have developed from astrocytoma tumours often have the IDH mutation, while *de novo* glioblastomas do not. If the tumour has the IDH mutation it is known as 9445/3. If it does not have the IDH mutation (known as IDH wildtype), it is called 9440/3. If doctors are unable to gather the data about the IDH mutation – say because a biopsy is not possible – it is called NOS, and the tumour is labelled and treated as if it *does* have the IDH mutation.

The main point is that certain treatments are considered to be more or less effective for 9445/3 compared with 9440/3. A full genetic picture means patients are given the treatment that is most likely to work for them, and which doesn't waste their time and energy or affect their quality of life unnecessarily.

One final example that will be relevant to glioblastoma patients. Some glioblastoma brain tumours have a gene inside them known as MGMT, and it is responsible for producing a protein also called MGMT. The protein helps to repair damaged DNA in cells, so protects cells from tumours. However, MGMT also helps cancer cells to repair themselves. If your glioblastoma has a large presence of MGMT proteins, then your chemotherapy of temozolomide is less likely to be effective. If you have low MGMT levels, then the chemotherapy can be more effective.

So the presence or absence of MGMT genes and proteins in your tumour cells is predictive of how effective temozolomide might be. Before you begin chemotherapy, your oncologist will want to determine the tumour's MGMT presence, so as to be able to plan whether to offer you temozolomide or not.

All this means that treatment for brain tumours had become super targeted. Sure, it's not a cure, but it allows better tailored and more appropriate treatment.

"Overall, it is hoped that the 2016 CNS WHO will facilitate clinical, experimental and epidemiological studies that will lead to improvements in the lives of patients with brain tumors," says the WHO paper.[40]

Or as Dr Kenneth Aldape neuropathologist at the Princess Margaret Cancer Centre at Toronto General Hospital told an American Brain Tumor Association webcast:

"The major change in the new update 2016 is that we have reinforced the importance of these markers by putting... into actual definition some of these entities. In part to encourage the use of them universally when possible. Also to really help us define on a precision medicine basis of these tumours. Some of which can look the same in the microscope that have different micro features. Potentially differences in responses to therapy."[41]

Why does genetics matter to patients?

Genetics are a relatively new development, in terms of power and information for brain tumour patients and their loved ones, where previously information was quite hazy, particularly around prognosis.

Previously tumours of very different types would have been grouped together, producing very rough statistics for age, side effects, treatment advice and survival times. Now, researchers can go back over old data and impose the new definitions. A brain tumour patient might have previously been given a prognosis based on the statistics for *all* glioma tumours. When all brain tumour types are grouped together, the outlook is relatively good: a mean survival time of around five years.

But that's to paint a false picture, because when the types of brain tumour are separated, the prognosis for different types of glioma can be radically different. For a low grade oligodendroglioma the median life expectancy is up to 14 years. Meantime, a high grade primary glioblastoma would be the opposite end of the scale. The outlier tumours at either end of the wide group were skewing the figures, creating a false middle.

But that's not all. If you further separate even those glioblastomas, this time at a molecular level, the rejuvenated data shows a significant survival time difference between patients with a glioblastoma IDH mutant tumour, compared with a glioblastoma IDH non-mutated (wildtype). The data also shows what proportion of glioblastomas are IDH mutant, and what proportion are IDH wildtype.

As an example, those with glioblastoma IDH mutations have an average age at diagnosis of 40 years. Meantime, the glioblastoma IDH non-mutated (wildtype) have an average age at diagnosis of 62 years. Previously, all glioblastoma patients would have been grouped together (at least as far as a lay reader is concerned) creating a skewed picture of average age at diagnosis.

Please do note that all of the above is my attempt to explain the genetic signatures of brain tumours from a layperson and patient's perspective, to a like minded audience. It is actually far, far more complicated than you can imagine, and if you go back to the source material I'm using it won't be long before your eyes glaze over. To patients and loved ones, I hope I have been able to simplify things enough to give you an impression of why this stuff is important. To medics and researchers, please excuse the blunt instrument I've taken to your painstakingly detailed work.

Dealing with death

"I AM 28 years old and find the support for young people pretty lacking, and dare I say our peer groups aren't the best equipped to deal with death! Nor our relationships in general. I don't think I've had a single frank conversation with anyone on the subject of my prognosis."
Jack Webb

I do not wish to linger too long on the subject of death and dying, but my inclusion of this chapter is in direct response to what I have experienced as a lack of information and reassurance from doctors, and from charities, about death and brain tumours.

While there is some material that deals with death, it feels that much brain tumour material is technical, it concentrates on 'survivorship', and it passes patients' loved ones onto more general bereavement resources once they have passed away.

It is, of course, important for patients and loved ones to continue to live, to attempt treatments and to make the most of what they have. Some call this 'fighting' or 'surviving', and in the cancer community in general there is an urge to 'give it all you've got', to 'try everything' and 'fight' every step of the way. This is useful language for many, and a perfectly reasonable response. But it can sometimes prevent us from also talking about death being okay: not everyone wins their 'fight', and dying is a natural conclusion to these types of brain tumour. Admitting death is probable, and preparing for it – whether a patient yourself, or caring for a loved one – is sensible, balanced and reasonable. It is certainly not 'giving up'.

On the brain tumour talkboards, as well as in my own conversations with patients and research from various brain tumour charities, the feeling is that doctors don't often seem very good at talking to patients about death. Family members complain that doctors had not used the words until perhaps a week or two before their loved one passed away, which made their death all the more shocking.

The medic's emphasis had always been on survival, trying new avenues. Only rarely would the doctor talk about the possibility of death, and provisions for it, towards the beginning of a patient's brain tumour journey. This has become known as a 'culture of cure' that is preventing serious discussion about quality palliative (end of life) care for brain tumour patients. The consensus among patients and loved ones certainly seems to be that they would welcome an earlier discussion.

What I share here, then, are some ideas and information about thinking about death, the process and the reality. You may of course find it too difficult to read and wish to pass over it, or you may find it the most useful part of this book. My aim is certainly not to tell any patients to give up, that they don't stand a chance. That's not true. Many high grade brain tumour patients do live long and well lives. Some may die from causes other than their brain tumours. And in the next chapter, we'll learn about how scientists are pushing survival times back and back and back, with new knowledge, treatments and interventions.

But there may be a time, whether prompted by your doctors or not, when you as a patient, or as a loved one, may wish to begin thinking about death. In most cases, brain tumours do offer patients a little time. Rare is the case of a patient being diagnosed and then passing away within weeks. Patients and loved ones have shared that they welcomed this time between knowing that the end was possible or even near, to the patient passing away. These kinds of brain tumours allow families and patients themselves to think about, prepare for and to some extent take control of their loved one's passing.

The more control and understanding that patients and their families have ahead of time, the more chance that patients will have what is becoming known as a 'good death'. One that is peaceful, to some extent in the manner of their choosing, and among those whom they most wish to be with.

> "I took advice from a friend of mine in the
> UK who works in a hospice. Their policy is
> that you don't tell the patient anything, unless
> they ask, and if they do ask, then you tell them
> the truth. I was always waiting for the moment
> when Sue would ask me about her prognosis
> but she never did. She became fixated on 'the

piece of paper' that would prove she was cured. On a few occasions, though, we would cry together. On one, she sobbed, 'Oh Jo, I'm in a right mess'. I think then the truth was beginning to hit her."

Joanna Waters, sister of Sue Rossides

The following are some of the ingredients that have emerged from talkboards, groups and my own conversations, as brain tumour patients' and families' ideals of a 'good death'.

Communication with medics

Patients and families can seek information from their doctor about the likelihood of treatment working, and the short and long term effects, so that they can weigh that against the perhaps short life that a patient has. Though there are medical ethics and legal issues to deal with too, doctors should be aware that some families would rather a shorter, more comfortable move towards a patient's final weeks, days and hours, than a frantic, seemingly endless and ultimately fruitless mission to keep a patient alive for just one more month. What are our limits for pain and distress? Where does the patient and their family draw the line between a dignified passing, and one they would consider undignified? Patients and families would benefit from this discussion.

A dying plan

Many parents draw up a 'birth plan' for when we come into the world, outlining their ideal emotional and physical state for when they give birth. It does not always go exactly to plan, but it is an ambition to work towards. Why should we not begin to draw up a similar plan for our passing away? Central to the discussion a patient and their families might attempt to have is: What is our vision for a good death?

The kinds of questions that might form this conversation include, if you could choose: Where would you like to die? Who would you like to have around you? What things would you like to say or do in your final weeks and days? Who would you like to see (and avoid seeing!) before you pass away? What religious or ceremonial rituals would you request for before and after your death?

The results of these discussions might be passed to doctors, religious figures, and wider family and friends to shape a kind of 'dying plan' for the patient.

Living wills

In most Western countries, a patient can draw up what has become known as a 'living will'. In the United States, it is called an advance directive and in Britain it is called an advance decision. (It doesn't apply in Northern Ireland).

They are documents that you draw up that outline the medical interventions you will allow and not allow, if you should become unable to communicate your wishes yourself.

For example, you can write into your living will that you do not wish doctors to artificially continue to keep your body alive, if there is no prospect that it will recover and function by itself. You might ask that you are not resuscitated if you stop breathing. You might request that if you are considered 'brain dead', your body is not kept alive unnecessarily. You might request your body is kept alive only so long as is needed to use your organs to assist someone else to live.

The possibilities are wide, and it is up to you – with advice from organisations and perhaps legal help – to consider the different situations doctors may find themselves in. If there is no clear answer for them in your documentation, doctors are in most cases obliged to try to keep your body alive unless instructed otherwise by someone you have appointed to make a decision for you (called in the UK a 'lasting power of attorney').

It should be noted that, for the most part, living wills are legally binding. As long as you are in sound mind when you write yours, and it is co-signed by a senior figure such as a doctor or lawyer, then a hospital doctor or oncologist would be acting unlawfully if they go against your wishes.

While doctors have a legal obligation to reduce your pain and discomfort, they cannot treat you without your permission if your advance decision says they shouldn't. Family members, including your partner or spouse, can't overrule your advance decision either. It's advised you speak to them about your wishes before and while you're writing up any advance decision.

Options for treatment, or withholding treatment, vary from country to country, but in brain tumours they are likely to include choosing not to treat infections such as pneumonia with antibiotics; choosing not to resuscitate you if you stop breathing; withdrawing an artificial breathing or feeding tube; and increasing doses of morphine or another drug.

However, you can override your own wishes at any time, simply by saying so (as long as you are regarded as having the mental capacity to make decisions on your own behalf). Note, in some countries you cannot ask doctors to 'switch off the machine' or give you overdoses of medicine that are certain to result in your death. In others, doctors may legally use your advance decision as a basis for their actions in these circumstances, but ultimately they will have the casting vote. Usually, they will go with your wishes unless there is reason to believe your wishes are not clear, or were not relevant to the specific circumstances.

You are strongly advised to contact an end of life charity in your own country, should you wish to consider writing a living will and appoint a lasting power of attorney, or equivalent, to look after your medical interests if you become unable to communicate them yourself.

Leaving a legacy

Death feels like the time to impart our wisdom on the world, however old we are. You may feel this is a good time to record – either in writing, by audio or video – some thoughts for your loved ones, particularly young children who might have to come to know you by what you leave behind. If you have no direct messages to leave, perhaps a short history of you, your values and your thoughts about the world might be welcomed by those who love you.

A friend whose father died suddenly while he was young said one of his biggest regrets was that he had no physical remembrance of his dad, except a few faded photographs. Sometimes, he couldn't even remember what he looked like. This is of lasting sadness to him.

For the sake of any children or partner you may have, it may be worth considering what you could leave. Since my diagnosis, my wife has written an almost daily diary about me and my relationship with our children, and she's taken to frequently videoing and photographing us as a family simply doing the kinds of things that families do. We both want our children to see the things we did together, how I spoke and what I looked like.

The American Brain Tumor Association received a presentation from Alan Carver, neurologist at the Sloan Kettering Cancer Center. He recommends some questions that might help to create such a legacy:[42]

• Tell me about your life history. When did you feel most alive?

• Are their specific things that you would want your family to know about you, to remember?

• What are the most important roles you have played in your life?

• What are your most important accomplishments?

• What do you feel most proud of?

• Are there particular things that you feel still need to be said to your loved ones?

• What are your hopes and dreams for your loved ones?

• What have you learned about life that you would want to pass along?

Wills

This is something we all should be doing from the moment we start earning money, owning anything worth money, and certainly if we have children or dependants.

Of course, my wife and I didn't have wills, despite our house, our children and my relatively expensive collection of bicycles. The diagnosis prompted us to finally get our wills drawn up. A will is simply a legal document that outlines what should happen to your assets and your dependants in the event of your death. You and your partner, if you have one, should have a will drawn up for each of you.

A solicitor friend of ours offered to do ours for free; it was something he could offer that was concrete and helpful. In fact, it's very possible to draw up your own will. You can download templates from the internet. Our wills described what should happen to our assets – our money, our home etc. – in the event of our deaths. They also described what should happen to our children if we both, for any reason, became incapable of looking after them.

You'll also need to appoint an executor of your will, basically someone who is responsible for making it all happen. Again, this may be something concrete and useful a good friend will be willing to do – particularly to take any stress off a partner. You are advised to check the legislation regarding wills and probate (the distribution of assets) in your own country.

All of these are difficult decisions, but once they have been written into your will it somehow eases the burden. You'll know that the major piece of paperwork is in place, not just if your brain tumour ends your life, but if you die or become incapacitated for any other reason too. A few decisions, a bit of paperwork, a relatively small financial outlay, and it's done.

Practical affairs

For any of us, there are practical affairs that we may not until now have ever thought of. For me, that included the fact that I owned my own company. Who would run it when I'm gone? Where should any money go? Would there be tax to pay? Who would pay it? Who would close down the company?

What practical affairs do you think you might need to put in order? Perhaps you own your own property, or have a flat that you let or a holiday home. Perhaps you run an organisation or charity, or have investments and multiple bank accounts that need sorting out.

If nothing else, we all have a series of passwords and account numbers for our computers, bank accounts and online presences. Will you ask someone to take care of those kinds of practical arrangements for you, or just leave them to sort themselves out?

Another aspect you may wish to consider is funeral arrangements. These are likely to be closely aligned to your values, religious beliefs and culture. You should note that unless you state, probably in writing, what you wish to happen at any funeral or memorial service, then it will be for your family members – or for the relevant authorities – to arrange proceedings on your behalf. And they may not chime with your own wishes.

Only you and your closest loved ones know what you're really like, and what you'd really want after your passing. It may seem morbid to be planning your own funeral, but some may find it cathartic – a job done – to consider music and atmosphere, who you would like to speak, the kind of service you would like, and what you would like to happen to your body when you have passed away.

Bucket list

A bucket list is an informal name for a list of things you might like to do or achieve before you die. Lots of people have bucket lists in their minds, even if they haven't any health problems at all.

Do you want to go to Las Vegas or see the Grand Canyon? Have you always wanted to try skiing or cave diving? Have you always promised to get round to learning Spanish or get serious about your photography or painting?

These are the kinds of things people put on their bucket list. As someone diagnosed with a life limiting disease, you may find drawing up a bucket list something useful. It may give your life a focus, finally encouraging you to do the things you'd always wanted to do.

Others may not have a bucket list or anything like it. Indeed, some may feel pressured to draw one up when it isn't something they really want to do.

When I've been asked – particularly by people I don't know well – what's on my bucket list, I've felt uncomfortable. What may or may not be on my bucket list – if I had one – might be an incredibly personal matter. You'll want to make your own choices about whether to draw one up, and what it contains.

> "I know in the end it'll kill me, but then something will. I think that I will think about it more when it gets closer to the end than right now. I am lucky that I do not have to worry about having children. I would have loved to have a couple but maybe in the end it is best that I couldn't."
> Richard Stevens

Duncan Weaver's daughter was just two and a half years old when his consultant told him and his wife that his low grade tumour had transformed, and he now had a dangerous anaplastic astrocytoma.

As reluctant as they were, it was time for Duncan and Loes to allow themselves to doubt he would be around to see Tess grow up.

Duncan began to make videos for young Tess. Mostly he talked about what he was like, about their family, and that he was very proud of his daughter. He was desperate that Tess would grow up knowing her Daddy. Duncan made four videos over the year, then Loes took over, making regular videos of Tess and her father together, laughing, chatting at lunch or simply playing on the sofa.

In September 2016, doctors had told the couple there was nothing else they would be able to do, except make Duncan as comfortable as possible.

It was that same day that Loes told Tess what was happening to her father. It was a beautiful sunny afternoon, and Loes took Tess to the beach so Duncan could have a rest at home. Previously she'd been too young, so Duncan and Loes hadn't told her anything about his illness. To her, Daddy having a bad leg and arm was normal. It was a matter of fact not difference that Daddy sometimes brought her to school on a mobility scooter. She would show off her mode of transport with pride.

But Loes felt the time had come to stop pretending that Daddy would be better again soon. She asked Tess if she'd noticed how Duncan's arm and leg had got worse lately, and how tired he had become.

"Yes, of course," she replied, like it was the most normal thing in the world.

Loes told her that Daddy's body was slowly breaking down, like a broken dolly can sometimes break bit by bit, until they don't work at all anymore.

That would mean Daddy would be dead, and that it would be just the two of them from then on.

At first, Tess looked at her mother thoughtfully. Then she asked if Daddy would become a star in the sky. Loes told her daughter that Daddy would be the brightest star of all, and that he would always be with them.

"Well, that's okay then," Tess said, turning back to her sandcastle.

> "After temozolomide hadn't worked, I was briefly switched to PCV treatment, but then only to Lomustine [one of the drugs in the PCV regimen]. Halfway through the treatment time, when I was expecting just a minute or two with a registrar, my oncologist showed up. His comment was that all of the drugs I had been given had failed to work. He basically expressed his view that my brain cancer was no longer treatable, except with palliative care. We were devastated and cried all afternoon. I looked and felt good. To be told this completely out of the blue was a total shock."
> Graham Dunnett

Palliative care is a growing field. Even 10 years ago, the care of people who were given a terminal diagnosis and no longer receiving potentially life saving treatment was considered a social issue, rather than one that needed a medical input too.

Today, our attitude to death has changed and so has our attitude to palliative care. Hospitals and oncology departments now have palliative teams who oversee a patient's medical and pastoral transfer to wherever they would wish to spend their final months, weeks and days.

Where previously palliative care tended to mean moving a patient into a hospice, so that a hospital bed is freed up for someone else, now it is a discipline that seeks to look in a more holistic way at a patient and their family's needs.

How would they like to pass away? How can they be made most comfortable and as free of pain as they can be during this time? How can patients be assisted to achieve a degree of dignity and independence in their final months, despite their decreasing abilities?

If you are advised by your medical team that there is little else that can be done to treat your tumour, that does not necessarily mean the end of treatment unless that is what you want.

Medical palliative care is still an option: doctors may prescribe further radiotherapy, chemotherapy, and even carry out further surgery simply to make you more comfortable, or to help maintain some of your motor or cognition skills, even if it will not extend your life.

You may also be offered medication, pain relief, physiotherapy, walking aids, complementary therapies and other measures to attempt to maintain your quality of life for as long as possible. There is likely to be a time when you are passed from your usual medical team to palliative care specialists, but this will be because they are best placed to meet your needs.

Within around the last six months of your expected life, you may be offered the opportunity of hospice care. This may take place in a building or hospital like complex where nurses and doctors are on hand continuously for those approaching the end of their lives. Or you may wish to request 'hospice at home'. In the latter, a palliative nurse specialist will visit regularly at home, to give you treatment and to give your loved ones some respite from your care, and to continuously assess your health.

The Neuro-Oncology Gordon Murray Caregiver Program at the University of California points out that while palliative care is common among cancer patients, some aspects are particularly of note for brain tumour patients.[43] They include a patient's degrading cognitive and motor skills, their sensory abilities, delirium, changes in behaviour, increased seizures, physical and mental problems with eating and drinking related to nausea and ability to swallow, and fatigue. Brain tumours can also affect bowel function.

What you are able to receive will obviously depend on the country in which you live, and the insurance, health and social care system that operates there. More and more health insurance providers are now including paying for quality palliative care as part of their offer. For those less well off, charities may be able to provide funding or hospice places for those with terminal brain tumours.

The World Health Organization now considers a 'good death' as a human right, and as such has drawn up nine principles for patient care at the end of their lives.

Palliative care, says the WHO, "improves the quality of life of patients and their families facing the problem associated with life threatening illness, through the prevention and relief of suffering by means of early identification and impeccable assessment and treatment of pain and other problems, physical, psychosocial and spiritual."

According to the WHO principles, palliative care:

• Provides relief from pain and other distressing symptoms;

• Affirms life and regards dying as a normal process;

• Intends neither to hasten nor postpone death;

• Integrates the psychological and spiritual aspects of patient care;

• Offers a support system to help patients live as actively as possible until death;

• Offers a support system to help the family cope during the patient's illness and in their own bereavement;

• Uses a team approach to address the needs of patients and their families, including bereavement counselling, if indicated;

• Will enhance quality of life, and may also positively influence the course of illness;

• Is applicable early in the course of illness, in conjunction with other therapies that are intended to prolong life, such as chemotherapy or radiation therapy, and includes those investigations needed to better understand and manage distressing clinical complications.

Do doctors and nurses, or even hospices, always get death right? No, of course not. But it is very good to have some principles to work from in order for patients and loved ones to know what they ought to expect, and which they can urge professionals to work towards.

With family, friends and loved ones, good palliative care – along with lots of communication – is the ideal situation in which to experience the 'good death' we perhaps all hope for.

After Duncan's doctors had done all they could, Loes and their family established hospice care for him. In the Netherlands this is provided by volunteers. An oncology nurse would also visit their home regularly, to help with dressings and medication, but also to share a cup of coffee and talk about whatever.

The most important message she shared was that Duncan should not waste energy worrying about getting dressed or up for the day, getting up and down from the sofa, or making food. Almost any activity left Duncan short of breath and she wanted him to take it easy, save his energy for when his wife, daughter and any visitors would call round.

Not long after – swallowing his pride and finally admitting to the loss of independence it would bring – Duncan allowed the hospice to install a hospital bed downstairs in their house. To him it felt like a defeat, but the positive aspects quickly showed themselves. He could control the bed himself, and didn't waste most of his energy for the day just coming downstairs. He could sit more comfortably in bed, and more easily get out and onto the mobility scooter so the family could head to the beach for an ice cream for Tess.

Soon, though, Duncan's ability to get out and about reduced further. He could still get out of bed, and even managed trips out on his mobility scooter a couple of days a week. But he could only do very short stretches before he needed to rest and sleep again. Communication became difficult, as his speech deteriorated. After three more weeks, he could no longer form sentences. Loes had an instinct for what he was trying to say, as partners do, but friends and family were often at a loss. Their sometimes hamfisted attempts to talk to him only resulted in confusion and frustration on all sides. Not long after losing the ability to speak clearly, Duncan started to struggle with understanding what was being said to him as well. He did not lose understanding completely, but he needed to hear simple and practical things, always said in short sentences.

It was as if he needed all his concentration to just be able to think, which meant he couldn't be around his happy, chatty, noisy daughter for too long. As for any father, guilt and sadness were his natural response. But he was happy that she would still climb up in bed with him, read him books, and Tess would tell her dad about school and sing songs.

What happens at the end?

One of the things I most desperately wanted to know after diagnosis was what the process of dying from a brain tumour would actually look like. Would it be painful and long drawn out? Would I suddenly keel over one day without expecting it, or would I know weeks before exactly how long I had left?

Of course, every patient's experience is different. Researching this book, I have heard the occasional terrifying story of a patient in great pain and distress at the end of their life. But that has been far from the majority.

In most cases, patients have either experienced death in the circumstances they had hoped for, or have drawn up some kind of 'dying plan' which they hope to be able to achieve – obviously, as long into the future as possible.

What is most reported is that a patient passed away

at home, peacefully and among loved ones. I've received many more stories than I can share here of poignant moments of togetherness, when a patient has passed from life to death without drama or panic.

Of course panicked and unexpected death does happen in brain tumours, but with anaplastic astrocytoma and glioblastoma brain tumours it appears clear that those who pass away more frequently experience a gentle and painless death.

The pressure in the brain may lead to sickness, weakness and some pain, but you will be given very effective medication to ease this. Most likely, it is then a case of the patient sleeping more and more, eventually for days at a time, until they eventually do not wake up again.

Peter Black, brain surgeon and author of *Living With a Brain Tumor*, writes: "It may help to consider that often when a person with a brain tumour is nearing the end of his life, he is less afraid than he was early on, when the brain tumour was diagnosed.[44]

"Symptoms that we often see at this stage are difficulties with speech and swallowing, lethargy, incontinence, and difficulty with walking. A person may become increasingly withdrawn or lapse into a coma... In the very last days, the person's breathing may be laboured, but in this phase she will be unconscious, so he or she will not be afraid. Often a person's transition to death is peaceful."

The Neuro-Oncology Gordon Murray Caregiver Program publishes a very good booklet about palliative care, including an extremely detailed section on what to expect in the last few days and hours of a brain tumour patient's life, with advice on how loved ones might cope.[45]

It too predicts that many brain tumour patients will gradually sleep more and more, and fall into unconsciousness. But it also says that patients can experience very slow breathing, weakness, decreased appetite and thirst, some pain and distress.

Poor ability to clear liquid on the lungs, coughing or repeated swallowing is another signal that the body is closing down, as is loss of bowel control. Typically, the guide says, these symptoms are more distressing to the family than to the patient who may be unaware by this point.

The guide urges families to continue to talk to and touch their loved one, including them in their conversations and considerations: "We don't know for sure what unconscious patients can actually hear, but it is prudent to presume that the unconscious patient hears everything. Families should talk to the patient as if he or she were conscious. Try to create an environment that is familiar and pleasant. Surround the patient with the people, children, pets, objects, music and sounds that he or she would like."

> In some ways, it was a blessing that Sue's comprehension vanished and she spent her last few months with no fear, and with very little pain. It's the most one can hope for. I feel no guilt. I know that I did everything I possibly could do."
> Joanna Waters, sister of Sue Rossides

> "George's breathing had changed. I went into George's room and could see he was trying to open his eyes. He had not been able to open his eyes since mid January. I said, 'oh you are

trying to open your eyes, you are my superman after all the drugs they have given you this morning'. I think George was trying to say goodbye and gifting me one last look into his beautiful eyes. My Georgie took his last breath. I cradled his head in my arms and told him over and over how much he was loved and will always be loved, how very brave and courageous he was."

Jane Cooke, mother of George

It had been a busy day for Duncan, Loes, Tess and the family. The couple's parents had been around for tea and cake. Duncan had been able to sit up on his bed listening to the olds chatting away. Something in the conversation caused Loes and Duncan to look away from the gathering and into each other's eyes.

"I remember, we just looked at each other for a long time across the room. It was a look that said it all: how much we loved each other, how proud we were of our daughter, how much we loved our family, and how much we were going to miss each other," says Loes.

That night, a bump in the night had awoken Loes and she'd come down to check on her husband. Duncan was lying on the floor. His eyes were open and he saw her come in, but he didn't move and he didn't try to speak.

Loes pulled him over, propped him up against the sofa, while she reached for her phone to call for help. She talked to the home care nursing team who said they would be on their way. She also called their local doctor, who was unavailable, but soon after called back. The doctor asked some more questions, like whether his muscles were tensed.

"When I said they weren't, she told me to just hold him and talk to him lovingly, because this could well be it.

"It wasn't until that moment that I realised that he was dying, that this really was it. So I just held him tight, told him how much Tess and I loved him, and that we were going to be okay. Then his breathing just got slower and slower. Until eventually, it stopped.

"All I can say is that I am eternally grateful that I woke up that night, that he saw me come in, knew I was there with him, and that I was holding him in my arms when he died."

Tess was upstairs and fast asleep when her father died. She had remained asleep as the nurses had come, and the local doctor had arrived and confirmed Duncan's death. He had passed away quickly and painlessly, she said, an impingement on the brain stem that would have closed his body down in a matter of moments.

Loes had never planned for Tess to see her father after his death, but as the undertakers came to take his body away she changed her mind. It wasn't right that his daughter would wake up in the morning and Daddy would no longer be there.

"So, slowly I woke her up, and asked her if she remembered how I had told her that Daddy's body was slowly breaking down, until it was completely broken. She nodded and I told her that was what had happened. That Daddy was dead now.

"I asked her if she wanted to go downstairs and give her Daddy a kiss before they took him away, which she did. Duncan was lying flat on the floor, with a duvet over him as though he was asleep. Tess went into the living room, walked up as normal, kneeled down to him and gave him a big love and a kiss. We then went upstairs again. And the undertakers took Duncan away."

Nearly three years after her mother had been diagnosed with a glioblastoma brain tumour, Lian Davis noticed her mum was spending more and more of her time asleep.

She kept asking Gillian why she was being so lazy, but often her mum would just smile or swear in a cheeky way at her daughter. Lian had long stopped Googling brain tumours, so didn't recognise long periods sleeping as a sign of the body closing down.

"One day we could barely wake her," says Lian, "and we called the nurses." They came out and said she had a bit of an infection, but I could tell by the looks the nurses were giving each other that they knew. They'd come to love my mum and could see how loved she was.

"That day we called an ambulance as we wanted her infection treated. At hospital they put in a drip, but told us it probably wouldn't do much. That was when I knew. Mom hadn't woken up for 24 hours. I cried as I hugged her and said: 'We all love you so much Mom.'

"It was then she said her last words. I'll never forget: 'I love you 'n all.'"

Gillian went into a coma for almost 48 hours. They played her reggae music, knowing she was listening, perhaps remembering how she used to love dancing. When her mum died, it was nothing like Lian had imagined it would be. There was a moment of noisy breathing, and then simply quiet.

Peace washed over the whole room.

Living after the death of a loved one

I do not aim to counsel the bereaved, nor advise them on how to live when their loved one has died from a brain tumour. I am far from qualified to do so, and there are those – both authors and individuals – with much more experience and confidence to do so than I.

What I do hope to do is highlight one or two of the common experiences of those left behind after a patient has died specifically as a result of their glioblastoma or anaplastic astrocytoma. My aim is to demonstrate that what you may be feeling is not unusual or unnatural, and that you are not alone. Charities in particular, and the support groups and talkboards that they host, will offer much stronger support than I can here. But I suspect you may find the following themes reflected wherever you look.

Blame

Brain tumours are still a very poorly understood form of cancer. In fact, many of us affected by them experience an almost perverse sense of jealousy that brain cancer seems to come so low down the pecking order and popularity stakes, compared, for example, with breast, lung or testicular cancer.

Brain cancer is far harder to detect, not least because there is no lump that can routinely be checked for. The symptoms of a brain tumour – headaches, poor balance, nausea, seizures – so closely mirror those of so many other conditions that it is no wonder they are routinely overlooked. As I wrote earlier in these pages, doctors do miss brain tumours simply because they are much more likely to be something less serious.

But we cannot help but apportion blame,

particularly when a loved one dies. Doctors should have done more. They should have detected it earlier. I should have listened harder when my partner told me of his symptoms. We shouldn't have passed off Dad's wobble as just getting old and frail.

In the fog of grief, we're bound to question who is to blame, even if we conclude it is ourselves, so we can create a target for our pain.

Anger and blame are a natural part of the grieving process, and I do not wish to dismiss them – and indeed sometimes doctors do behave negligently. But perhaps time will heal the anger and blame, along with coming to a full understanding that brain tumours have no cause. Nothing could have prevented a loved one's glioblastoma or astrocytoma, and very little could have changed the eventual outcome. There is no definitive evidence that earlier diagnosis of these tumours leads to longer overall survival times. They remain the most stubborn of cancers in terms of survival rates. Most often, there is no fault to be laid. You certainly are not to blame for your loved one's brain tumour. You couldn't have done more, even if looking back you feel like you could have.

> "Who knows how long George had the tumour. I look back and think it might have been there a long time. When he was complaining of neck pain and I was saying 'Oh, its all that time you are playing Playstation hunched over'. Or the headaches, sometimes after a night out with friends that cleared after a couple of paracetamol. Or the bad back he once complained of when he was about 16 and we went for therapy. Could all

that have been tumour then? I feel I let George down as I did not know and I am his mum. I should have known."

Jane Cooke, mother of George

Relief

Brain tumours can break apart relationships, putting even the strongest bonds under pressure. As we have seen, some relationships do not survive the pressure and there should be no blame or feelings of guilt attached to them.

Personality change among patients, combined with the unexpected role change from partner to carer, can make even the most solid relationship turn to little more than day to day functioning. If a partner has become stressed or depressed, verbally or even physically violent, or if their needs are so great that their daily care has become hard to deal with, then it is no surprise that a carer may feel a sense of release when their partner dies. It is perhaps worthy of note that I sometimes half heartedly welcome the idea of dying myself, because I seek relief for my partner who has at times had to take on so much of the family burden, including my depression and personality change. It may be that your own loved one will feel the same feeling of relief at finally being able to give you a break.

None of us should feel guilty about these feelings of relief. They are a natural part of being human. Feelings of gladness for ourselves and grief for the patient who has recently died will be bittersweet. We may be sad for their passing, but their death releases them, you and your family from suffering, burden and uncertainty.

Those who have faith may perhaps draw strength from the tenets of beliefs here, while others may gain a sense of life and the universe continuing on its path.

Rapidity

In some cases, glioblastoma brain tumours can wreak damage with extreme rapidity. It can sometimes be a matter of months, even weeks, between diagnosis and death. This scenario does not give the patient or loved ones time to prepare for the future that is hurtling towards them, as doctors do all they can to extend a patient's life.

The nature of such cancers is that they will stun and shock a loved one. They may have spent the last month in panicked hospital wards and consultants' offices, rather than even considering the idea of death or grieving.

Those who go through this rapid process can expect to feel little but numb after a loved one has passed away, and surprise those closest to them with functionality and lucidity.

In those early weeks, it will be the hardest battle to come to terms with the idea that, though you were only together seemingly a few days ago, your loved one is not coming home. Eventually, shock will give way to grieving. Loved ones and family will need mutual support as the realisation sinks in and life changes beyond measure.

Grief while living

Brain tumour patients and loved ones report feelings of complete grief even during the time they have remaining. They then feel guilty about these emotions, because shouldn't they be making most of the time they have left? As time ticks along, you want to seize every second together with joy and positivity, yet you can't get out of bed, can't stop crying, can't pull back the curtains to allow the last rays of sunshine in.

Once again it is natural to grieve while your loved one is still alive, and indeed it can be cathartic for you to grieve together. Where possible, you may find it helpful to talk about your memories and emotions, the best times you had together, the things that made you happy about each other.

You could talk too about grieving for what you may not be able to do: see a child or grandchild grow up, visit far shores, or simply grow old together. You may decide to write final letters to each other, take lots of video and photographs, and give gifts that reflect your relationship. Many patients and loved ones report feelings of satisfaction about being able to actively grieve together with the person they have had to lose.

Expectations

Death of a loved one from whatever cause will create a wide range of emotions: relief, guilt, grief, anger, sadness and happiness, often wrapped up into a messy ball. There is no need to attempt to unwrap this ball in any rush, nor feel guilty that you have not yet brushed yourself down and begun to get on with your life.

As the recommended *Palliative and End-of-Life Care for Patients with Brain Tumors* guide puts it: "These are all normal things to feel. There is no right or wrong way to express and deal with all these emotions. Give yourself the permission and latitude to experience whatever emotions you may be feeling. It is not your fault. Do not feel guilty about your emotions, asking for help, or asking questions and wanting to be prepared for the end of life."[46]

Clinical trials and latest research

"I STILL FIND reasons to be cheerful. I try to have at least one big thing to look forward to after each round of chemo, to keep up my morale on the bad days. I love to be on the move, so usually it's a day trip, a short holiday, a visit back to the UK to see my family. But every day there are things to be cheerful about. I love going for walks in the countryside, or in the city, meeting up for a catch up with friends. I know it's a cliché, but I certainly appreciate the small things in life much more than before."
Calum Wright

Though this book necessarily has a negative overall outlook, things are slowly getting better for brain tumour patients. First, diagnosis is getting quicker and symptoms are being better recognised. That means brain tumours are being caught earlier. That means a better chance of a good quality of life for patients living with a brain tumour.

Second, after many years of brain tumours being the 'Cinderella' of cancers, left alone and relatively unconsidered while their sisters like breast, lung and blood cancer got all the attention, authorities are now recognising the underinvestment in brain tumour research. In even the last five to 10 years, this realisation has led to new funding being pushed towards brain tumour research and some notable successes in understanding how the tumours work, and what might be done to slow down or even stop their progress. Even in my five years of diagnosis, I've seen new possibilities emerge that were not on the table when I was first told.

Because of their nature – particularly that they grow in a very difficult place to reach, and within areas that control our bodies – brain tumours will always be an intractable problem. But the challenge is on and it looks like the scientists are slowly gaining on many cancers, and in brain tumours they have come a very long way. This offers reasons to be cheerful.

Clinical trials

Not only does all of this mean that patients with glioblastoma and anaplastic astrocytoma tumours might benefit from new developments coming on stream even as I write, but that there are also more opportunities than ever for patients to participate in clinical trials that may help them – and others that come after them.

Whether the clinical trial is a success or not, medicine will have learned something, it will have moved on, and the growing canon of knowledge about brain tumours will benefit patients in the near and distant future.

If you have come to the end of standard treatment, it is very possible you will be offered the chance to enrol in experimental treatment, or be asked to join a clinical trial. Indeed, you might be asked to join a clinical trial before you are given any treatment.

A clinical trial is any kind of research study that seeks to determine whether a particular course of action – say a series of chemotherapy, a diet, or a surgical technique – is effective in achieving proposed goals. Usually this would be improved health outcomes. In brain tumours, that might be regarded as a longer life span, a longer progression free period before a tumour reoccurs, or a better (measurable) quality of life even if ultimate lifespan is not extended.

The question, for example, might be: If I give the patient this form of chemotherapy, will it be more successful in keeping the patient alive, but with the same or less toxicity to the patient as the current standard chemotherapy?

Clinical trials are far from restricted to drugs though. They might involve surgical techniques, exercise regimes, radiological procedures, changes in care protocols, and many other things.

It is also worth noting that not all clinical trials have the direct aim of improving or extending life, though that would be the overarching aim in the long term. A trial might simply be to see if a glioblastoma cell behaves in a particular way; say whether it repairs its DNA or not, given the presence of a certain chemical. Or a trial might be to see if a certain drug works the same as another, but produces more tolerable side effects.

These trials may seem like small fry, but their implication is that scientists discover more about how brain tumours are formed, or function under particular conditions. That then guides future research that might be better used to treat them.

In short, not all clinical trials are 'potentially life saving treatment' as the more sensationalist newspapers would have it. Those who join clinical trials may not be looking for a miraculous cure, but to contribute a very small part to the medical knowledge of why malignant brain tumours do what they do.

Of course, there *are* amazing, ground shifting trials, and some of them are astoundingly successful, but these would be the exception rather than the rule.

There are a couple of other important points to consider, if you are asked or inclined to participate in a clinical trial. Your doctor will usually want to exhaust all of the known effective treatments with you first, as their obligation is to try what has been known to work with tumours of your type. If they do not think a treatment has a chance, they should not be giving it to you at all. That is when they might ask if you are interested in participating in a clinical trial. You will be provided with very clear information about the treatment under investigation before you decide to participate, and you will be monitored closely.

But participation is not a right. Different doctors, hospitals and cancer centres, as well as universities, have their own research projects, with their own funders, and very strict criteria for participation. Moreover, if you have a health insurer they may decide that they are not willing to pay for your participation in a clinical trial. Your having a glioblastoma or anaplastic astrocytoma does not put you to the front of the queue. Researchers need participants who fit specific criteria, so that their research is sound and addresses the questions they are asking.

In the same way, you may be unable to participate in a clinical trial because – ironically – you have received treatment for your brain tumour. A trial may be designed, for example, only to treat people for whom temozolomide has never been used. If you have had the drug, you will not be eligible.

It is worth noting that many clinical trials need to have a control arm. That means that some patients receive the treatment under research, but others (randomly selected) receive nothing, or a 'placebo' – a fake form of treatment. You will not know which arm you are participating in. This is because researchers need to know whether it really is their treatment that is causing the improvement or change, or whether merely participating in the research is having an effect.

This 'placebo effect' is very real, and it is important to design trials that account for it. The outcome, of course, is that you may be signing up for a clinical trial that you believe may contribute to your life chances, when actually you're receiving a sugar pill while someone else on the trial is receiving real drugs.

Finally, you can participate in a clinical trial but actually play no real role whatsoever. In fact, you probably already are. Research is taking place all the time that looks back on statistics, on patients, their MRI images, their blood, their biopsies and diagnoses. Researchers are looking at new things they have discovered about brain tumours, and then projecting that new information back onto data collected over the last decade or more in order to prove or test it. Past statistics can prove newly proposed theories.

Before my biopsy, I gave permission for my blood, samples of my brain tissue and my MRI images to be kept, as it were, 'on file' for future brain tumour research. I'm not sure if this literally means there are pieces of my brain in a fridge somewhere. What I suspect is that full medical, epidemiological, chemical and biological records were taken in great detail, as well as photographs, so that my data can be used in research projects, along with the data from thousands of other brain tumour patients. Various brain tumour centres and universities have established 'brain banks' of information and samples that can be used in ongoing research in this way. Not very glamorous, but absolutely essential for analysing huge numbers of patients. And that's what great scientific research is all about.

Clinical trials are very strictly managed, and are overseen by senior research boards and ethics committees. The World Health Organization (WHO) has a strict protocol for clinical trials, for biomedical dugs, treatments and other interventions:

I. Testing the intervention in a small group (20-80 participants) to evaluate safety, a safe dosage and to identify side effects;

II. Clinical trial among several hundred patients, to determine efficacy and further evaluate safety;

III. Study among hundreds, preferably thousands of patients, comparing the intervention to the standard of other experimental treatments, collecting detailed information about adverse effects;

IV. Study of patients after a product, intervention or drug has been marketed and put on general release, particularly monitoring any adverse effects.

It is a shame to report that many brain tumour trials do not reach stage III, either because drug interventions are found to be too toxic or not effective enough to pursue. Often patients don't live long enough to complete the trial, or there are insufficient patients undergoing the trial to draw sufficiently solid conclusions from stage II. In many cases, patients aren't even asked to participate in a trial.

This is why researchers in the brain tumour field are increasingly working on a worldwide scale so that larger numbers of participants can be included in studies. The WHO runs its own International Clinical Trials Registry Platform, which attempts to gather together all medical trials taking place, to enable researchers to gain from and contribute to others' research, and to prevent unnecessary duplication.[47]

Unfortunately, funding is an issue in most clinical trials, with universities, funders, drugs companies and governments often looking for quick wins in the research they support – something that is rare in brain tumour science.

If you wish to join a clinical trial, your first port of call should be your own brain tumour doctor, surgeon or oncologist. They may know of suitable trials for you. Your own country may also host its own registry of cancer related clinical trials, and it is worth using their search engines with the words 'glioblastoma' and 'astrocytoma' to see if there is anything locally that you can become involved with.

The WHO registry can be searched for brain tumour related trials.[48] In the UK, the most comprehensive registry is run by Cancer Research UK,[49] though the UK Clinical Trials Gateway may be of use because it uses worldwide data sources.[50] The

US equivalent of the same database, also claiming to source from many dozens of country's trials, is ClinicalTrials.gov.[51] The American Brain Tumor Association (ABTA) runs the TrialConnect service, which matches patients with clinical trials that may be appropriate for them.[52]

All of them have more information about how clinical trials work.

If you are considering enrolling in a clinical trial, you will need to do so through your medical team. ABTA offers some important questions to ask about the trial before participating:

"When evaluating a treatment, ask your doctor how the recommended treatment will affect your prognosis. What are the expected benefits of this treatment? What are the risks? What quality of life can you expect during and after the treatment? If this is an investigational treatment, how many patients with your tumor type have received this treatment, and what were their results? Is there a placebo control arm as part of the study? Is this covered by insurance and research funding?"[53]

Finally, a note on 'trials' and 'clinical trials'. Patients and loved ones should take note that in cancer, there is a huge amount of 'trialling' taking place. But not all of it is of a medical nature.

There are many non-medical treatments, complementary therapies and experimental 'cures' on offer. They sometimes masquerade as 'trials', for which patients have to pay in order to participate. I can do little but urge caution here, as it is a rough terrain to negotiate, particularly when we are desperate. If you come across a trial that makes claims to cure or prevent cancer in the brain, or elsewhere, you should always consult with your medical practitioner and oncologist about the biological plausibility of the treatment, as well as the legitimacy of any claims it makes.

It is also worth exercising caution about claims that a certain treatment or diet is being offered to patients, based on even scientific trials currently taking place. Too often patients are urged to buy a particular substance, or buy into a treatment plan, because scientific researchers are having 'promising results in trials' of this substance, or something relating to it, at a respected institution. The key word here is 'promising'. It indicates the trial, even if it is legitimate, isn't yet complete. No conclusions have yet been drawn. Just because a treatment is being tested does not mean it definitely works.

Cutting edge research

> "I try not to worry about the future too much, but it is inevitable that it sometimes sneaks into my mind. At the beginning of this journey, I didn't dare to forward plan. The MRI scans essentially dictated my life. I wouldn't make any plans and if someone asked me to arrange something, I would be very vague about it. Now, I am getting better at looking to the future with less fear."
> Calum Wright

As I write, there are some very real developments in brain tumour research that could make a difference to you as a patient now, and to glioblastoma and astrocytoma patients in the future.

This may be in terms of overall lifespan, in terms of preventing reoccurrence after initial treatment, in reducing side effects of the tumour or its treatment, or improving quality of life.

Thankfully, by its very nature, research moves faster than any single writer or book can keep track of. For the latest news on the most cutting edge discoveries and research on glioblastoma and anaplastic astrocytoma, you are urged to consult your local charities and brain tumour centres, who will be tracking new developments very closely and will most likely be involved in the funding of them.

What I aim to outline here are some of the most recently emerging, promising areas of research and treatment. I have already covered the rapid development in 'biomarkers' in brain tumours; that is, the genetic signatures of brain tumours and their influence on effective treatment. Naturally, researchers are also attempting to improve the type and combination of drugs used to treat brain tumours, including introducing chemotherapy that has been found to be useful in other cancers. This is slow and painstaking work, but it is going on every day and hardly ever makes the headlines.

In the following, I aim to give an indication of what else is going on, why, and what difference it is having or might have in the future. Some of the following will be out of date by the time you read it, some of it may have failed, some of it may have become standard practice. That's the pace at which brain tumour research is moving just now, and that can only be a good thing.

Immunotherapy

This is one of the most exciting areas of brain tumour treatment research. It must be said that the treatment is still very much in the testing phase, and is not yet considered a standard treatment. But immunotherapy is being given to some suitable anaplastic astrocytoma and glioblastoma patients with a view to extending and improving their quality of life.

It is by no means considered a cure, merely another tool in the armoury of short term treatments for brain tumours. In the very long term, however, immunotherapy could lead to much wider options for treatment of brain tumours and this has generated lots of interest among clinicians, patients and the media.

Unlike traditional chemotherapy, in which the drugs you take attack tumour cells, immunotherapy drugs aim to make your own immune system more effective at 'finding' and destroying cancer cells. Cancer cells in the brain can avoid the normal function of our immune system by 'disguising' themselves or making themselves 'invisible'. The result is that the cancer is free to grow into brain tumours.

Immunotherapy works in a number of ways, and each technique is being researched. More research is looking at how the different types might work together. In one area, immunotherapy drugs attach molecular 'signals' to cancer cells, revealing them to the immune system where once they were 'invisible'. The immune system is then able to find and destroy the cells.

In another area, immunotherapy drugs boost the immune system by giving the immune system a virus. The virus can kill cancer cells, and also gives the immune system the ability to kill cancers that have previously evaded it.

What is most important about immunotherapy is that it assists the immune system to find and attack cancer cells. Like all cells, cancer cells can experience DNA disruption, which can mean they change. Because they grow quickly, a changed DNA that makes it more likely to survive means those cancer cells can very quickly multiply, creating very resilient tumours. If a tumour changes so that some of its cells become resilient to a particular chemotherapy drug, those resilient cells will regrow into a chemo-proof new tumour. This is sometimes why chemotherapy isn't effective.

By concentrating not on the tumour cells, but on the immune system, immunotherapy gets around this evolution tendency in cancer. The immune system is re-armed, able to attack any kind of cell that isn't behaving as it should, thus making cancer cells more vulnerable. Unfortunately, like other therapies, some patients are inherently resistant to immunotherapies and some patients who initially respond to immunotherapy eventually acquire resistance.

Currently, immunotherapy is being offered to some glioblastoma and anaplastic astrocytoma patients for whom the first lines of defence have failed, or when a tumour has reoccured. Because it still requires very strong chemotherapy drugs, immunotherapy can have a very toxic effect on the body. In some cases, the side effects are so severe that immunotherapy has to be stopped.

Oncolytic virus therapy

A type of immunotherapy, this was once thought to be the next big thing in glioblastoma treatment. This technique – which involved using existing viruses such as herpes to tackle brain tumours – was found to be far less effective in humans than it had been in mice. Human brains too easily washed away the virus, it was found, which at least vindicates the importance of the clinical trial system for testing treatments. However, potential still exists in attempting to 'infect' brain tumours by keeping the virus inside and close to the tumour site by encasing what is left behind after tumour in a gel that is teeming with the virus.[54] Research is ongoing, but it does show the novel and 'out of the box' approaches that scientists are taking to tackle brain tumours.

Surgery techniques

One of the most promising developments in surgery techniques for gliomas is what has become known as the 'pink drink'. It's something scientists are trialling right now across the world and are having some significant success with.

One of the key problems about brain tumour surgery is that you need to remove as much as possible to make a significant difference to both the quality of life and the life expectancy of patients. And if you can remove tumour cells but not the healthy tissues around them, you're less likely to damage parts of the brain that make the body work. As Dr Colin Watts, a consultant neurosurgeon at the University of Cambridge who is at the forefront of this research, puts it: "In certain areas of the brain, such as those controlling movement, a millimetre can make the difference between a patient being disabled, or being able to walk out of hospital."[55]

In addition, tumour cells don't often look much different to healthy brain tissue and that some cells are bound to remain if they're lurking in and around creases in the brain. This is where the pink drink comes in. The pink drink (which is called 5-ALA and isn't actually pink) can make brain tumour cells appear a glowing pink under ultraviolet light. That means a brain surgeon, armed with an ultraviolet torch, can distinguish better between the tumour and the healthy brain tissue around it.

That means more brain tumour can be taken out. Surgeons can also see bits of tumour lurking in nooks in the brain they wouldn't otherwise have seen. And they can avoid cutting away bits of the brain that aren't glowing.

The science is very new, but progress is so far very encouraging. If you can stomach it, there are some amazing videos of the pink drink in action during brain surgery on YouTube.[56]

There is also a non-surgical aspect to this research. Dr Watts is seeking to determine how brain tumour cells behave in different areas of a tumour. The 5-ALA dye is allowing him and his researchers to identify areas in tumours of different intensities and malignancies, to sample them accurately, and then to look at the biochemical profile of the different areas with more or less identified malignancy. It's all part of understanding what makes particular brain tumour cells malignant, compared with other brain tumour cells. Identifying the differences between them could lead to better targeted treatment.

Crossing the blood-brain barrier

The brain is fiercely protected by our bodies from infection that is carried in the blood by a complicated 'blood-brain barrier' that allows only certain types of molecules through and into the brain. Drugs are treated as foreign molecules by the blood-brain barrier, so many are unable to pass. Over 95 per cent of drugs do not show useful activity in the brain and many show poor penetration of the blood-brain barrier.[57] Unfortunately, this means that many of the chemotherapy drugs used quite successfully for other cancers around the body can't be used to tackle brain tumours.

An increasingly strong arm of research is looking at how to develop or 'edit' chemotherapy and other drugs so that they are not prevented from crossing the blood-brain barrier. In some cases, this involves attempting to get the drugs into tumour 'sinks' within the mass itself, so that the drug can proliferate.

Likewise, researchers are examining how they might temporarily 'switch off' the blood-brain barrier to allow chemotherapies that have been proven to effectively kill cancer cells to work on brain tumours. Some of this research is the stuff of sci-fi, with researchers creating nano particles (like ultra tiny robots) and coating them with chemotherapy drugs, before opening a gap in the barrier using ultrasound, so the particles can be guided by magnets into a tumour.

A yet third area of research is to explore the gamut of drugs that do cross the blood-brain barrier, to see if any of them might have a tumour cell killing capacity. Or whether those drugs can be 'edited' to have a chemotherapy effect.

Active research is looking at certain anti-depressants and drugs for erectile dysfunction, for example, since they are known to cross the barrier and have direct effects on the brain. Other research has examined the use of anti-malarial drug chloroquine – which also crosses the blood-brain barrier – as a 'booster' for conventional brain tumour chemotherapy.

Enhanced imaging

The accurate imaging of brain tumours is a vital tool in the oncologist and neurologist's kit for identifying brain tumours, and predicting their future behaviour. Indeed, medical experts in brain tumour imaging are able to look at the proliferation of blood vessels in brain tumours through 'dyeing' the blood before MRI scans, allowing them to better observe their growth rate and proliferation. Some research is showing that blood vessel proliferation can be an accurate predictor of transformation of low grade brain tumours to high grade, which means earlier action can be taken to treat them.

Imaging techniques like Diffusion Tensor Imaging (DTI) can show up where tracts of brain tissue are being pushed out of the way by a growing glioma, thereby showing their extent and size. Over a period of time, mapping of the movement of white matter can show the growth and infiltration of the tumour. One study found that the less disrupted the white matter around the tumour, the better the patient's life expectancy.

A project based at the Department of Neurosurgery at Cambridge University is looking at how advanced imaging methods, including DTI, can be used to predict where a glioblastoma tumour is likely to grow back before any treatment is given.

"There has been a lot of research looking at how using advanced imaging methods can tell you more about a tumour, but only a handful have shown how you might use them to change how you treat a patient," says Dr Stephen Price, a consultant neurosurgeon at the University of Cambridge. "Once we developed a method of identifying tumour regrowth with a high degree of accuracy, we could look at changing what we operate on or what we treat with radiotherapy."

The researchers' most recent data suggests that removing more of these early identified areas leads to improved patient survival and delays progression.[58]

Understanding brain tumours

Much of the research in brain tumours currently taking place is not about how best to treat them, but about how and why they form in the first place. This is particularly concentrating on their genetic makeup.

The aim of this research is to determine the nature of brain tumours, so that better treatments can be developed that get right to the heart of what makes these types of brain tumours so malignant.

If you like, scientists are going right back to basics so that brain tumours can be tackled on their most basic molecular level. It may seem strange that money is being spent looking at the nature of brain tumours, rather than trying ever new treatments in the hope of slight improvements in life expectancy. Certainly, if you or a loved one has a glioblastoma you may decry this kind of research as useless to you.

The truth is, though, that the treatment you may have, or be about to receive, is a direct result of just this kind of research many years ago. It is only by slowly understanding the genetic markers of anaplastic astrocytomas, for example, that it has become clear in what circumstances temozolomide will be effective.

That research money is perhaps better spent on the fundamental details than throwing money at a handful of possible approaches to tumours in the hope that one will work.

One particular international project in this area is a good example. The Institute of Cancer Research (ICR) in London, along with partners in Europe and the USA, has been examining the changes that take place in cells that appear to cause brain tumours.[59] They have concluded that some 26 different 'malfunctions' in a person's genes are required for a glioma to develop. Taken together, these malfunctions affect how brain cells work in a number of ways, such as how brain cells divide, how their DNA repairs itself, the life cycle of cells, how proteins are produced and how they respond to damage.

One of the research team's aims was to detect how many of these DNA malfunctions might be hereditary. The scientists were also able to identify the malfunctions that were, and were not, likely to influence whether the glioma tumour would be a glioblastoma. The research was the work of an international consortium of researchers, and was the largest study to date of malignant brain tumours looking for genetic markers.

"This research... in the future could allow doctors to identify a subset of people who may be at risk, and lead to the discovery of much needed targeted drugs," says The Brain Tumour Charity in the UK.

Afterword

EVERY FEW DAYS while I was writing this book, a new video popped up on my Facebook feed that made me smile more than the usual guff you get.

Mostly it was cobbled together shaky footage, but the backgrounds and the landscapes were unmistakeable and beautiful. It was Antarctica.

In one, James Campling and his dad delight as they dangle their freezing cold feet into one of the southern-most moving streams in the world. Not long after, James headed alone into the freezing wastes of Antarctica. In another Facebook film we see penguins up close; one more has him mucking around in a canoe, ploughing through mini icebergs floating on the freezing cold sea. I imagine a whale might pop over the horizon at any moment.

Other videos showed slightly warmer climates, as James traveled south through Patagonia towards his final destination. It appears to be the trip of a lifetime and the landscapes are astounding.

Afterwards, James returned to England just in time

to see a close friend complete the London Marathon in aid of the UK charity Brain Tumour Research.

A couple of days later, now over a year since his initial diagnosis, James Campling emailed me out of the blue. He'd had a seizure just hours after he'd returned from Antarctica, the first since emerging from his operation. A few days ago, he'd been for the results of his latest MRI scan.

"It wasn't really until I got to the waiting room that I started worrying, and then there was no escaping it. Finally, I was called through," he wrote. "My oncologist showed me the scan, and the previous scan. It's small, but it's there. The tumour has come back. I tried hard not to cry. I thought if I did give into this it'll be the start of depression. So I maintained the stiff upper lip the British are famous for."

James went into surgery once more, again at Oxford's John Radcliffe hospital. He then began the familiar to and fro of trying to balance seizures and mini strokes, steroids, diet and drugs. Soon after, he felt well enough to attend a job interview.

In his latest communication with me, he talked yet again of his true passion. Travelling. He might not be able to be as ambitious as he has been in the past, and his plans might not be as long term as they once were. But he's hoping to at least head back to India at some time, he says wryly.

"Every time I try to go to Australia overland," he jokes, "this bloody brain tumour seems to get in the way.

"Yes, I am going to die," he signs off. "But not yet."

* * *

I want to extend my grateful thanks to everyone who has been involved in the writing and researching of this book. In a very real sense it 'belongs' to the many voices included inside it, as well as many other brain tumour patients and their loved ones whose stories I have read, gained from and been moved by. I'm only sorry I couldn't include more stories and more words of wisdom.

In particular, I would like to mark the contribution to my own life of my good friend Marie Hunter who passed away from her anaplastic astrocytoma early in 2017. She was my partner in crime in brain tumours, we followed each other's journeys closely, and her sad death finally confirmed my need to write this book. I miss her and she has been in my thoughts every time I've opened my word processor to work on these pages.

I also wish to offer my thanks to each of the brain tumour patients and loved ones who shared their stories with me and allowed me to use their quotes. In particular, I am in debt to Loes Hartman-Weaver and Lian Davis who were willing to break their hearts even further in order to tell their stories. In many cases, their stories were already so beautifully written and sentiments so clearly expressed that I did little more than a light edit of their words. Thanks are also due to Duncan Weaver, for sharing his life and story with me in my previous book. Thanks too for the constant updates from James Campling. Good luck James with every journey you make, wherever they may take you.

Thank you to Toni Sidwell at The Brain Tumour Charity for providing support and a very detailed medical check for the whole book; any remaining errors are my own. Thanks to my editor Barney Jeffries, and to my wife Sarah Mole.

You will notice that I have not included a resources section in this book. That is because this is a very fast moving field, and any publications I may suggest will very quickly become out of date.

Instead, I urge you to ask your oncologist, clinical nurse specialist, or seek out your local brain tumour and cancer charities to ask for their publications or further recommended reading.

The internet can be good and bad for research on brain tumours: proceed with caution, and always check with your medical team before taking any action as a result of something you have read or seen online.

If you have found this book useful, moving, informative or otherwise, please help others affected by brain tumours to find out about it. I would be very grateful if you would post about this book in your social media, share it with brain tumour support groups, and please write an honest review on Amazon or any other review platform.

Thank you,

Gideon Burrows
Belfast, September 2017
gideon@ngomedia.org.uk

Brain tumours: Living low grade

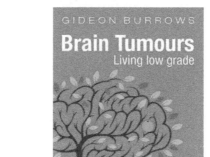

Slow growing brain tumours change lives forever.

This readable and moving non-technical guide is about living with a low grade tumour, a diagnosis given to thousands of people every year.

Featuring dozens of personal testimonies from those dealing daily with the impact of their tumours, this book offers information, support and reassurance for those with a low grade brain tumour, their family and friends.

ISBN: 9780955369575

This Book Won't Cure Your Cancer

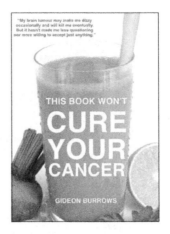

When Gideon Burrows was diagnosed with an incurable brain tumour, he found himself in the cancer twilight zone: a place where hope and wellbeing are exalted, and where truth and rationality are sometimes optional extras.

It's a world where the dying are always bravely battling, survivors are venerated and where charities and wellness gurus are beyond criticism. It's a place of miracle diets, self healing and positive thinking.

When there are so many contradicting opinions and so much background noise, how do you separate the sane from the sound? How do you make decisions that are wise rather than wishful thinking? This book challenges the very foundations of how we respond to the disease.

ISBN: 9780955369599

Notes

[1] American Brain Tumour Association, *Glioblastoma and Malignant Astrocytoma* (PDF) (Accessed 29 March 2017)

[2] Cancer Research UK, http://www.cancerresearchuk.org/health-professional/cancer-statistics/statistics-by-cancer-type/brain-other-cns-and-intracranial-tumours (Accessed 27 March 2017)

[3] David N. Louis et al., *The 2016 World Health Organization Classification of Tumors of the Central Nervous System: a summary* Acta Neuropathol (2016), 131:803–820 (Accessed 26 May 2017)

[4] National Cancer Institute, SEER Programme, https://seer.cancer.gov/statfacts/html/breast.html (Accessed 18 August 2017)

[5] The Brain Tumour Charity, *Glioblastoma* (PDF) (Accessed 10 April 2017)

[6] American Brain Tumor Association, *Glioblastoma and Malignant Astrocytoma* (PDF) (Accessed 29 March 2017)

[7] *Public Health England, Routes to diagnosis 2015 update: brain tumours*, http://www.ncin.org.uk/view?rid=3177 (Accessed 15 August 2017)

[8] Inside Radiology, *Gadolinium Contrast Medium (MRI Contrast agents)*, https://www.insideradiology.com.au/gadolinium-contrast-medium (Accessed 10 April 2017)

[9] The software I use is called OsiriX. A patient version is available free for the Mac operating system at http://www.osirix-viewer.com (Accessed 10 Feb 17)

[10] *Living With a Brain Tumour*, Peter Black (Owl Books, 2006) p.

148

[11] The Brain Tumour Charity, *Glioblastoma* (PDF) (Accessed 10 April 2017)

[12] National Comprehensive Cancer Network, *Brain Cancer – Gliomas, Version 1. 2016* (PDF) Accessed 18 April 2017)

[13] Braintstrust, http://www.brainstrust.org.uk/advice-coping.php (Accessed 19 April 2017)

[14] The Brain Tumour Charity, *Losing Myself, 2016* (PDF) (Accessed 13th April 2017)

[15] The Brain Tumour Charity, *Personality Changes and Brain Tumours*, https://www.thebraintumourcharity.org/understanding-brain-tumours/living-with-a-brain-tumour/side-effects/personality-changes-and-brain-tumours (Accessed 13th April 2017)

[16] Ownsworth T, Goadby E and Chambers SK (2015), . Frontiers in Oncololgy. 5:33. doi: 10.3389/fonc.2015.00033

[17] American Brain Tumor Association, http://www.abta.org/brain-tumor-information/symptoms/headaches.html (Accessed 13 April 2017)

[18] The Brain Tumour Charity, *Losing Myself, 2016* (PDF) p.10 (Accessed 13th April 2017)

[19] *I had a black dog*, Matthew Johnstone (Robinson, 2012). View the videos at https://www.youtube.com/watch?v=XiCrniLQGYc and https://www.youtube.com/watch?v=2VRRx7Mtep8 (Accessed 18 April 2017)

[20] I'm grateful to Epilepsy Action in the UK for much of the detail in this section: https://www.epilepsy.org.uk/info/seizures/focal-seizures, (Accessed 10 March 2017)

[21] Charles J. Vecht et al., *Seizure Prognosis in Brain Tumors: New Insights and Evidence Based Management*, Oncologist. 2014 Jul; 19(7): 751–759, https://www.ncbi.nlm.nih.gov/pmc/articles/PMC4077452 (Accessed at 5 May 2017)

[22] The Brain Tumour Charity, https://www.thebraintumourcharity.org/understanding-brain-tumours/living-with-a-brain-tumour/side-effects/epilepsy-seizures-and-brain-tumours (Accessed 10 March 2017)

[23] John Hopkins Medicine, http://www.hopkinsmedicine.org/neurology_neurosurgery/centers_clinics/epilepsy/seizures (Accessed 10 March 2017)

[24] The Brain Tumour Charity, *Diet* (PDF) (Accessed 13 April

2017)

[25] American Brain Tumor Association, *Diet and Nutrition for Brain Tumor Patients,* presented by Hannah Dalpiaz, RD, LDN, CNSC. Original webcast 30 March 2017, http://www.abta.org/brain-tumor-information/anytime-learning (Accessed 13 April 2017)

[26] *This Book Won't Cure Your Cancer,* Gideon Burrows (ngo.media, 2016)

[27] American Brain Tumor Association, *Ketogenic Diet For Brain Tumor Patients,* presented by
Leonora Renda, RDN. Original webcast 8 October 8 2014, http://www.abta.org/brain-tumor-information/anytime-learning (Accessed 13 April 2017)

[28] The Brain Tumour Charity patients and carers' support Facebook page, with permission of the author (Accessed 23 March 2017)

[29] The Brain Tumour Charity, *Losing Myself, 2016* (PDF) (Accessed 15th August 2017)

[30] The Brain Tumour Charity, *Mummy has a brain tumour,* https://www.youtube.com/watch?v=r9YTKO7-9aw (Accessed 14 April 2017)

[31] Macmillan Cancer Support, *Talking to Children and Teenagers When an Adult Has Cancer.* Information also available at http://www.macmillan.org.uk/information-and-support/coping/talking-about-cancer/talking-to-children/advice-on-talking-to-children-about-cancer.html#19687 (Accessed 14 April 2017)

[32] American Brain Tumor Association, *Glioblastoma and Malignant Astrocytoma* (PDF) (Accessed 15 March 2017)

[33] Cancer Research UK, http://about-cancer.cancerresearchuk.org/about-cancer/brain-tumours/survival (Accessed 15th March 2017)

[34] The Brain Tumour Charity, https://www.thebraintumourcharity.org/understanding-brain-tumours/getting-a-diagnosis/prognosis/prognosis-specific-brain-tumours (Accessed 15th March 2017)

[35] American Brain Tumor Association, *Glioblastoma and Malignant Astrocytoma* (PDF) (Accessed 15 March 2017)

[36] Cancer Research UK, http://about-cancer.cancerresearchuk.org/about-cancer/brain-tumours/survival (Accessed 15th March 2017)

[37] National Comprehensive Cancer Network, *Brain Cancer – Gliomas, Version 1. 2016* (PDF)

[38] The NICE guidelines and workflow can be viewed at https://pathways.nice.org.uk/pathways/brain-cancers (Accessed 22nd May 2017)

[39] David N. Louis et. al., *The 2007 WHO Classification of Tumours of the Central Nervous System*, Acta Neuropathologica, August 2007, Volume 114, Issue 2, pp 97–109, https://www.ncbi.nlm.nih.gov/pmc/articles/PMC1929165 (Accessed 26 May 2017)

[40] David N. Louis et al., *The 2016 World Health Organization Classification of Tumors of the Central Nervous System: a summary* Acta Neuropathol (2016), 131:803–820 (Accessed 26 May 2017)

[41] American Brain Tumor Association, *New Global Classification of Brain Tumors*, presented by Kenneth Aldape MD. Original webcast 26 October 2016, http://www.abta.org/brain-tumor-information/anytime-learning (Accessed 20 March 2017)

[42] American Brain Tumor Association, *Understanding Palliative Care*, presented by Alan Carver, MD, Memorial Sloan-Kettering Cancer Centre. Original webcast 29 March 2013 http://www.abta.org/brain-tumor-information/anytime-learning (Accessed 26 June 2017)

[43] Michael Cohen et. al., *Palliative and End-of-Life Care for Patients with Brain Tumors*, Neuro-Oncology Gordon Murray Caregiver Program at the University of California, San Francisco.

[44] *Living With a Brain Tumour*, Peter Black (Owl Books, 2006) p. 226

[45] Michael Cohen et. al., *Palliative and End-of-Life Care for Patients with Brain Tumors*, Neuro-Oncology Gordon Murray Caregiver Program at the University of California.

[46] Michael Cohen et. al., *Palliative and End-of-Life Care for Patients with Brain Tumors*, Neuro-Oncology Gordon Murray Caregiver Program at the University of California. The guide advises loved ones seeking the help of a doctor if they are still grieving after six months. For some loved ones, the grief is a form of post-traumatic stress disorder.

[47] WHO International Clinical Trials Registry Platform, http://www.who.int/ictrp/en (Accessed 21 April 2017)

[48] WHO International Clinical Trials Registry Platform search engine, http://apps.who.int/trialsearch/default.aspx (Accessed 21 April 2017)